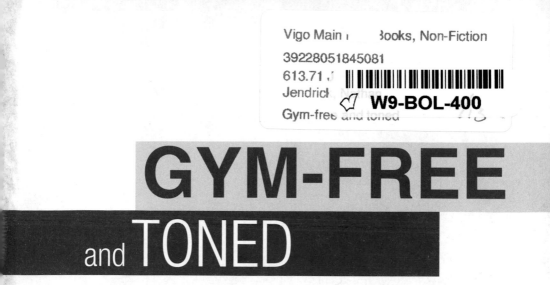

GYM-FREE
and TONED

WITHDRAWN

GYM-FREE
and TONED

Weight-Free Workouts
That Build and Tone

Nathan Jendrick

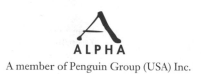

ALPHA

A member of Penguin Group (USA) Inc.

ALPHA BOOKS

Published by the Penguin Group

Penguin Group (USA) Inc., 375 Hudson Street, New York, New York 10014, USA • Penguin Group (Canada), 90 Eglinton Avenue East, Suite 700, Toronto, Ontario M4P 2Y3, Canada (a division of Pearson Penguin Canada Inc.) • Penguin Books Ltd., 80 Strand, London WC2R 0RL, England • Penguin Ireland, 25 St. Stephen's Green, Dublin 2, Ireland (a division of Penguin Books Ltd.) • Penguin Group (Australia), 250 Camberwell Road, Camberwell, Victoria 3124, Australia (a division of Pearson Australia Group Pty. Ltd.) • Penguin Books India Pvt. Ltd., 11 Community Centre, Panchsheel Park, New Delhi—110 017, India • Penguin Group (NZ), 67 Apollo Drive, Rosedale, North Shore, Auckland 1311, New Zealand (a division of Pearson New Zealand Ltd.) • Penguin Books (South Africa) (Pty.) Ltd., 24 Sturdee Avenue, Rosebank, Johannesburg 2196, South Africa • Penguin Books Ltd., Registered Offices: 80 Strand, London WC2R 0RL, England

Copyright © 2012 by Nathan Jendrick

International Standard Book Number: 978-1-61564-209-0
Library of Congress Catalog Card Number: 2012941773

14   13   12   8   7   6   5   4   3   2   1

Interpretation of the printing code: The rightmost number of the first series of numbers is the year of the book's printing; the rightmost number of the second series of numbers is the number of the book's printing. For example, a printing code of 12-1 shows that the first printing occurred in 2012.

Printed in the United States of America

Publisher: *Mike Sanders*
Executive Managing Editor: *Billy Fields*
Senior Acquisitions Editor: *Tom Stevens*
Development Editor: *Jennifer Moore*
Senior Production Editor: *Janette Lynn*

Copy Editor: *Jaime Julian Wagner*
Cover/Book Designer: *Rebecca Batchelor*
Indexer: *Brad Herriman*
Layout: *Ayanna Lacey*
Senior Proofreader: *Laura Caddell*

For my son Daethan, who makes every day perfect.

Contents

1: Adopting a Healthy Lifestyle 3

Avoid Reality TV Shows 4

Getting Your Body Ready. 5

Simple Steps to Beginning a Healthy Lifestyle 5

Training Truths: Myth Busting 8

The Truth About Skinny Genes 10

Get Rid of the Junk Food. 11

Exercise 11

Get Enough Sleep 12

2: Nutrition: The Foundation for Everything 15

Diet vs. Lifestyle 15

The Trickle-Down Effect of Making a Change 17

Explaining Protein, Fats, Carbohydrates 18

Fibers, Fruits, Vegetables. 19

Water 20

Goal-Oriented Foods 20

Terrific Tea 20

The Benefits of Coffee. 21

Metabolism and Energy-Boosting Foods 22

Immunity and General Health-Boosting Foods. 22

Joint Relief Foods 22

Destroying Food Myths 23

Reading Food Labels 24

The Nutrition Panel 24

Front-of-Label Claims 26

How to Clean Up Your Cupboards. 28

Your New Nutrition Program 29

Finding Your Body's Caloric Needs. 29

Calories for Fat Loss 29

Calories for Muscle 30

Eat This, Not That. 30

Fighting Cravings 31
   Exercise 32
   Distract Yourself. 32
   Give It a Rest 33
   Drink Water 33
   Chew Gum. 33
The Costs of Healthy Eating. 33
Timing Is Everything. 37
   Breakfast 37
   Pre-Workout Meals 38
   Post-Workout Meals 38
   Last Meal of the Day 38
Your Personal Food Log. 38

3: Stretching Out 47

The Basics of Stretching 47
   Stretching Do's and Don'ts 48
   How Often? 49
   Safe Stretching 49
Upper Body Stretches 49
Core Stretches 56
Abdominals and Obliques 56
Lower Back and Hips. 57
Lower Body Stretches 61
Quadriceps. 62
Hamstrings and Glutes. 63
Calves. 66

4: Upper Body Training 69

Arms. 69
Chest 74
Shoulders 80
Back 86

5: Core Training 93

Why Train My Core?. 93
Core Myths. 94
Core Training 95
Abdominals and Obliques 95
Lower Back/Hips/Glutes 110

6: Lower Body Training 119

Quadriceps. 119
Hamstrings. 128
Calves. 134

7: Breathing Easier: Cardiovascular Exercise. . . 139

The Benefits of Cardio 139
Science-Backed Studies. *139*
What's Considered Cardio *140*
Target Heart Rate. *141*
Passing the Time. *141*
Getting Moving. 142

8: Ready-to-Go Workouts 155

How Much? How Often? 155
How to Use These Workouts 156
Workouts 157
Drop Sets, Supersets, Partials,
and Failure 176
Cardio Circuits 187

9: Beyond the Workout: After-Training Tips 193

Rest and Recovery. 193
When You Grow: The True Value of Sleep. *193*
The Risk of Overtraining *194*
Speaking of Supplements 194
Debunking Supplement Ads *195*
Supplements Facts *195*
Supplements That Work *196*

Protein Shakes: Casein, Soy, and Whey *197*
Concentrates vs. Isolates *198*
Timing *199*

A: Glossary 201

B: Food for You: Nutritious Recipes 205

Index 245

Introduction

Introducing the Gym-Free Mindset

Most people have their minds tied to an ideology of "I need a gym to get in shape." And whatever excuse they create—the gym is too expensive, too far away, too big, too small, has too many people who look at me—stops them from taking the steps necessary to getting in shape. To them, if there's no gym, there's no hope. But that just isn't the case. If you have the will and even a tiny open space in which to move around, you have everything you need. So get rid of the mental block—the excuses—and make up your mind that now is the time to get in shape and get the body, and the life, you have always wanted. It's a step-by-step process, but it all starts inside your head.

This isn't just a home workout book, this is an *anywhere* workout book. You'll find exercises you can do at home, in your hotel room, even at a playground! The only requirement to put the Gym-Free program to use is your own motivation. Wherever you find that—from within, from the mirror, from your kids—is up to you. But know this: nothing is stopping you from being happier, healthier, and more active than ever.

The Definition of Toned

The word *toned* means developed muscle that's visibly attractive. When people see someone with rounded shoulders, defined arms, and a slim waist, they think, "Wow, that person is fit. They're really toned." And it isn't a term that's reserved for a select few; it's one that the dedicated earned.

You may have heard people use *tone* as a verb, as in "I need to *tone* up." But there's no such thing as toning a muscle. You're either building muscle or you're losing it, but you can't *just* tone it. So to be clear: toning isn't a type of exercise. It is, effectively, the result of being lean and well trained.

Timeline for Results

Everyone wants results *now*. But people don't put on extra pounds overnight, so they can't reasonably expect to lose them overnight, either. Ultimately, the speed of your progress is going to depend on your goals, the time you have to train, and how much body fat you have to lose.

You've probably seen the infomercials that talk about how so-and-so lost 15 pounds in 2 weeks. And they may have, but it was probably very uncomfortable, and likely almost none of the weight loss was body fat. Instead, that person dropped a lot of water and was pretty dehydrated when standing on the scale. If you have a decent amount of body fat to lose, you can aim to shed 1 to 2 pounds of fat per week. This rate of loss is healthy, feasible, and focused on fat—not muscle.

Wherever You Are, There's Your Gym

A prime tenet of the Gym-Free movement is that wherever you are, you're able to train. If you're in the middle of nowhere, with absolutely nothing around you but solid ground and open air, you can get a great workout. However, there are things you can add that can assist you in increasing the variety of your training. Coming up I offer some suggestions, but keep in mind that even these items can be substituted in some cases with something as simple as a household chair. Be creative, be healthy, and be active!

Exercise Ball

An exercise ball is a great training aid for all sorts of exercises. They enable you to vary many standard exercises and add increased variety to core movements.

Average cost: $20-$25

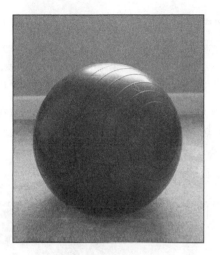

Stretch Cord

Instead of a huge row of dumbbells taking up all of the available space in your house, all you need is a stretch cord, which is also called a resistance band. With one of these handy workout aids you can do nearly all of the exercises you can do with traditional dumbbells, but stretch cords take up practically no space, are easy to take with you anywhere, and are inexpensive. If you're only going to have one piece of equipment, this is it.

Average cost: $9-$13

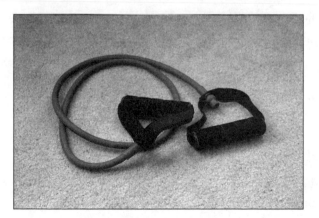

Medicine Ball/Dumbbell

Medicine balls are essentially heavy basketballs. They take up about the same amount of space but come in varied weights. A set, or even just one or more individual balls, make fun little additions to your training.

Dumbbells are also handy exercise tools; if you don't have room for that complete set of dumbbells, adjustable dumbbells are available, though these tend to be expensive.

Average costs: $8-$40 (medicine balls), $199-$399 (adjustable dumbbells)

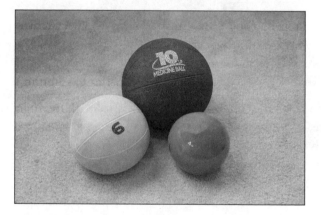

Apparel

Most people don't think of clothing as equipment, but it's vital you have adequate training apparel. Your clothes need to be comfortable but not too baggy. If you don't have the right clothing—even just a properly fitting t-shirt and pair of shorts—get them. You'll also want—dare I say, *need*—a good pair of shoes. I talk more about different types of shoes in Chapter 1.

Advantages of No-Gym Training

The Gym-Free and Toned lifestyle is a way to take control of your life and your fit future. As if you needed any other reminders, let's just take one last look at why this is the right move for you:

- No more watchful eyes.
- No more unsolicited advice.

- No more sweaty benches.
- No expensive monthly dues.
- No opening/closing hours.
- No closings on holidays.
- No limit to progress!

Acknowledgments

My never-ending thanks and love go out to my wife Megan and our son Daethan; to Don Anderson and Christena Warwick, to Michael Jendrick and, though best known as Stew, to Matt Nader.

For all of their hard work I thank my agent, Marilyn Allen, as well as Tom Stevens, Janette Lynn, Jennifer Moore, and the entire Alpha team who has made this project possible. It is only because of their watchful eyes and talents that this book has become the resource that it is.

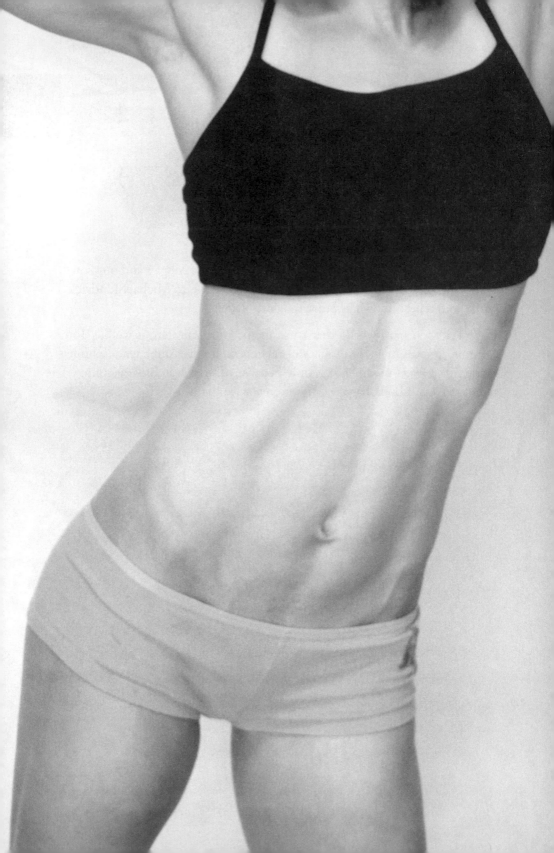

Adopting a Healthy Lifestyle

Diets don't work. Lifestyles do.

When well-meaning individuals say to themselves, "I'm going on a diet," they are already setting an end date for their efforts. And because diets aren't fun, they're surely planning to be miserable during that whole time. *Diet* is a term that exudes restrictions and hard work. People say, "I'm going to diet for twelve weeks, but in three months, I'll look great and it'll all be worth it!" But the issue is that when they go back to what they had been eating before—being off the diet—they'll also quickly revert to what they used to look like. So diets, as a whole, are just bad news.

Lifestyles, on the other hand, aren't hard work. They're simple. It's just living. You do what you do because that's who you are and you enjoy it. When you make fitness and health a priority, you make it part of your daily routine. It isn't limited in time or scope, and you'll always have it with you and, thus, always be making the right decisions and enjoying yourself. You'll also love what you see staring back at you in the mirror.

This book has all of the exercise and nutrition knowledge you need to get in the best shape of your life and maintain it for the rest of your days: exercises for every muscle group, heart-healthy cardiovascular routines, tasty meal tips, supplement advice, and more. It's all in here. But if you don't put it into action and use it, none of it matters. This is where the mental and physical aspects of becoming healthy come into play.

Avoid Reality TV Shows

You might be wondering why I'm talking about TV shows in a fitness book, but what we watch can have a big impact on our outlook toward ourselves and those around us. Shows about weight loss are big business. They draw sponsors who want to reach the huge audiences they achieve, and they present an image of what, supposedly, it takes to get in shape if you're overweight. Unfortunately, they're a horrible representation of both diet and exercise.

Why? Because the shows present unrealistic programs that normal people just can't follow. The contestants on these shows have chefs preparing their meals. Very few people in the world have that luxury. The people on the shows don't work while they're participating—again, a luxury few people have. So ask yourself, can you dedicate the time, money, and resources it takes to recreate the nutrition on these shows?

Next, the exercise programs the contestants are put through are ridiculous. The amount of weight they lose in such a short period of time can hardly be considered healthy. Rapid weight loss doesn't lend itself to long-term weight control. But if they do it slowly, it doesn't make for good television, and that's the main concern of this type of show. When certain shows pit contestants against one another on teams, thus making it one trainer against another with the winner determined by total pounds lost, all concern for the contestants' well-being goes out the window.

Contestants talk of working out for hours and hours a day. How many people have the free time to do what they do? The majority of people find themselves becoming overweight because work, family, and other life commitments take over, and eating right and working out take a backseat. So how realistic is it to think you can suddenly start working out four, six, or eight hours daily—and maintain it for the rest of your life?

The sheer volume of incidents where the medical staff of the show has to check on contestants should show you something is wrong with what they're doing. Most of the time, contestants on these shows are miserable. Becoming healthy shouldn't cause misery.

Being mentally sound and having a positive attitude is the number one factor in realizing you can take control of your life. Reality television convinces people that there is one way—their way—to get fit, and it couldn't be more wrong. So do yourself a favor and, when these shows come on, click them off. Let them be your cue that it's time to train, go for a walk, spend time with the family, or even just read a book. All are options that will surely be time better spent.

Getting Your Body Ready

You have to put everything in order to make things run as fluidly as they should. Surely, if you have nothing but Twinkies and snack packs in your cupboards, it's going to be difficult to get a healthy meal every few hours. Likewise, if you have too much clutter taking up your workout space, it's going to become more time-consuming and daunting to exercise.

Don't make your life more difficult than you have to; keep things orderly and available so that your new lifestyle is as easy and accessible as your old one.

Simple Steps to Beginning a Healthy Lifestyle

Follow these steps to help make your new, healthy lifestyle a reality:

1. Fix your kitchen

Because nutrition is the absolute foundation of a healthy lifestyle, you need to make sure your kitchen is in order. This doesn't mean you need to go buy fancy appliances or anything like that, but you should do a few simple things:

Throw out the junk food. Just get rid of it. Period. If it's not in your house, you won't eat it.

Keep your measuring cups handy. A lot of keeping your calories in check is simply thinking about how much you're eating. Most people can be just as satisfied eating $\frac{1}{2}$ cup of rice as a full cup, but their body doesn't tell them they're full until it's too late. The key to keeping your portions in check is to measure them out ahead of time. An easy way to do this is to organize the drawer your measuring cups—and teaspoons and tablespoons and the like—are in so they're easy to grab and use.

Buy some water bottles. If you don't have them already, pick up a few water bottles with the ounce notation visible on the side. Get at least one 20-ounce bottle for ease of travel and at least one 32-ounce bottle for workouts and other times when you can carry more fluids with you.

2. Fix your house

I'm not talking about finally repairing that leaky faucet. Instead, clear out a spot that's intended for you to work out. Whether that's the center of your living room or out on the back porch, clean it out and make sure it stays clear so it's ready when you are. Make this where you keep your equipment as well, if you choose to use any. The items suggested in this book include a resistance cord/band and an exercise ball (see later in this chapter).

Finally, make sure you have some workout clothes that are appropriate. Many people think they can just wear whatever's handy when they exercise, and you can, but you will want to be comfortable. If all you have are thick, hot, sweatpants and sweatshirts, you may want to find some more comfortable shorts and t-shirts.

3. Know what to eat when you're out and about: you can have a social life!

There aren't enough pages in this book to cover even a small number of the things people love to eat and drink when they're out with their friends, so this one is a simple homework assignment for you. If you hang out with friends at the bar or a favorite restaurant, do some research ahead of time and find out how many calories are in what you usually eat. If your standard fare is high in calories, find some things on the menu you enjoy that are more favorable to your waistline, and start ordering those items instead. Remember: just because it's a salad doesn't mean it's healthy. Dressings are, in fact, some of the most calorie-dense foods around.

Restaurant websites are a great resource, and if you're a fan of beer, for instance, you can run a simple internet search to find out how many calories are in your favorite pint.

Here's a tip to cut down on overeating while you're out: always ask the waiter to bring you a box with your food. Immediately put some of the food in the takeout box when it arrives to keep yourself from indulging too deeply.

4. Start recording your progress

A great trick you can use that will provide motivation in the weeks, months, and years ahead is to create an email address for yourself that you can send progress reports to. For example, you can create myfitnesslog@gmail.com and, every Monday, take a photo of yourself (even just from your phone) and email it to yourself. This is an easy way to keep tabs on your progress; you can log in to that inbox months later and look at how far you've come in such a short amount of time. You'll remind yourself how much better you're already feeling.

If you're pretty well organized without email, you can also take photos and store them on your computer or print them out instead.

5. Follow the principles of no-gym training

The Gym-Free training method doesn't require a lot of rules, but you do need to commit to a few key principles if you want to make it work for you. Here they are:

Make your training a priority. Your home, a hotel, or even your yard all make for convenient places to train. But it doesn't mean you should do random sets in between trips to the grocery store or episodes of your favorite show. Your training still needs focus, no matter how little or how much time you have and no matter where you are.

Embrace the effort involved in getting into shape. Training is not instant gratification. It takes work. Know that, embrace it, and be better because of it.

Set goals so that you train with a purpose. Don't just say, "I want to lose weight." Decide on the body you want so, as you go, you'll know you're making progress.

Training Truths: Myth Busting

Before delving any further into your fitness program, you should be aware of a handful of myths swirling around the concept of getting in shape. Here they are, in no particular order:

Myth #1: Training your muscles will make you huge. I wish I had a dollar for every time I heard a woman say, "I'm just going to do cardio because I don't want to get huge," or "I don't want to weight train because I don't want to look like a man."

Take heart: You won't get huge just by weight training. Putting on massive amounts of muscle takes many years, proper nutrition, and, a great help to that end, testosterone. Women have very little of the hormone most responsible for muscle growth and, as such, little worry of becoming bulky and overly muscular by training. But what you can expect by training are shapelier, more attractive muscles and a thinner, trimmer waistline.

Myth #2: Core exercises will burn ab fat faster. As mentioned earlier, there's no such thing as toning. As a result, there's no such thing as spot toning, which is the principle behind the long-held myth that doing a lot of crunches will get you a six-pack faster. This isn't the case, so please don't focus your workout around core exercises.

A lean midsection requires adequate training of the whole body *and* proper nutrition. Trust that you'll get there, and know that you'll have a whole lot more fun than just pounding out tens of thousands of sit-ups.

Myth #3: Cardio is better than weight training for burning body fat. There's this idea that, because you burn more calories running for an hour than you would doing push-ups or sit-ups over the same period of time (taking breaks between sets, of course), cardiovascular exercise is superior to muscular training for overall fat burning. This is not the case at all.

While it is true that running burns more calories than singular exercises, the difference comes into play during the times you're *not* training. Going for a run will burn calories while you're moving and even keep your metabolism elevated for a short period thereafter, but when your body has added lean tissue, you burn extra calories *all day long*.

Myth #4: No pain, no gain. Whoever coined the phrase, "No pain, no gain," when it comes to training probably lived a very uncomfortable life. Exercise shouldn't hurt, and while it's true you're going to feel tension and flexion on the muscles when training, there's no reason for actual *pain*. If you're feeling serious discomfort on that level, you need to stop, reassess your technique, and perhaps move on to another exercise altogether. Not every body is made for every movement.

Myth #5: Toning shoes help you burn more calories. Manufacturers have marketed toning shoes by saying that you will improve your health or fitness level simply by wearing them. Some are weighted while others are shaped in a particular way to supposedly increase muscle activation. The American Council on Exercise noticed, like the rest of us, that the claims of "Burn more calories just by walking!" and "Tone your legs and butt just by wearing these shoes!" were pretty outrageous. They paired up with a team of exercise scientists from the Exercise and Health Program at the University of Wisconsin–La Crosse, to give a few different types of toning shoes a thorough look.

Throughout their studies, the researchers found that *none* of the toning shoes showed a statistically significant increase in calories burned or muscle activation as claimed in the advertisements. Further, they found there's no evidence at all that toning or shaping shoes cause people to burn more calories or improve muscle shape, strength, or tone.

So what's the bottom line? Don't waste your money.

Myth #6: You should wear shoes with lots of heel cushion. Studies have shown quite conclusively that running without the heel padding typical of most athletic shoes puts much less physical stress on the joints of the feet, ankles, knees, and hips. As a result, shoe manufacturers have introduced minimalist footwear, which is basically nothing more than a thin barrier between your feet and the ground. The idea is to give your foot a more natural fall to the ground with each step. Two of the more popular minimalist shoes, if you can call them that, are Vibrams Fivefingers and FILA Skele-toe.

Studies have also shown that wearing this type of footwear improves the muscles in the feet. However, there are potential downsides. The most common side effect of minimalist footwear is inflammation in the lower body caused by doing too much too soon. By not working up to long-term use, overuse injuries can occur.

Keep in mind that any change in footwear is generally useless unless you also make sure that you're running properly. If you don't use the proper technique to put your foot to the ground time and time again, it makes no difference what's covering your toes.

Your goal should be to strike the ground first with the forefront of your foot, near the ball of your feet and not your heel. Striking the ground with your heel first places an incredible amount of force on your knees. Unfortunately, regular athletic shoes tend to make it more likely that you strike heel first rather than ball first! When you run barefoot, you're more likely to use the proper technique naturally.

The Truth About Skinny Genes

You can't choose your parents, so your genetic composition was pre-determined long before you could ever make a decision of your own. For some, that means they're shorter than they would prefer, or they don't care for the color of their eyes, or they have curly hair and have to work hard to straighten it (or vice versa). But those things don't affect one's health. A lot of your genes, though, *do* have direct correlation with health, and those are the important ones.

Unfortunately, people use the same excuse for their height as they do their weight. "It's not in my genes," they say. There's also a lot of talk about "big bones" or "I'm just meant to be big." It's all nonsense. No one is "meant" to carry around unhealthy levels of body fat. It's a personal choice, and it's something that can be changed—no matter what your genes are like—with hard work and discipline.

Everyone knows a person or two who seem to be able to eat anything they want without ever putting on a pound. The truth is that, yes, they have a natural, genetic advantage in that department by having a faster metabolism. It is what it is. Often times though, those same people have a tough time putting on muscle mass because of that same metabolism that helps keep body fat off. In turn, someone who may be prone to putting fat on easily may be able to build lean tissue just as well. It's important to understand that whatever your strengths and weaknesses are, they're all you've got and you have to deal with them. Fortunately, with a little educational reading—such as this book—you can also learn and understand a few things you can do to maximize your own genetic make-up.

Researchers out of Massachusetts General Hospital have said that half of a person's predisposition to weight is built into their genetic make-up. That makes any opportunities we have to alter these genes that much more important. What you eat, how often you're exercising, and how much you're sleeping, are just a couple of things you can change right now to improve yourself.

Get Rid of the Junk Food

For many people, their desire to eat junk food is an addiction. And the addiction grows from one food to the next—the more junk they eat, the more they want. The body then starts releasing massive amounts of insulin, which promotes fat storage, and the vicious cycle repeats itself.

Most people can—after some quality time spent on a healthy lifestyle plan—enjoy the occasional treat and have no issues. But you have to be very real with yourself and be honest and analyze how you react when you do this: Can you just stop at one cookie or a couple of squares of chocolate? If not, you need to remove the temptation to eat junk food by taking it out of your house. It isn't necessarily a will-power thing; you're not weak, your body and brain just don't handle it well. So if you need to take a step to prevent overeating of junk food, by all means give your shelves a thorough once-over and get rid of all the bad stuff for good.

Exercise

Researchers have found that the expression of "fat genes" in the body can be reduced simply by exercising. In fact, exercise has such a powerful effect on the genes that it can reduce their effect by a third. This means that, while you may be predisposed to gaining weight easier or losing fat less quickly than others, by getting up and getting active you're changing the way your body processes food and you're changing your metabolism. For everyone, exercise is beneficial, but for people with specific fat-centric genes, you're really going above and beyond when you train consistently.

Get Enough Sleep

There's a direct correlation to how much sleep you get and how much your genes contribute to your overall body weight. The more you sleep, the less effect those genes have; consequently, the less you sleep, the more effect your genes have on your waistline. And in this fast-paced world of ours, that's bad news. But it's all the more incentive to ensure you get the rest you need. When you're getting inadequate sleep, you're also more prone to overeating due to a decrease in hormones that cause you to feel fuller.

Shoot for 7 to 9 hours of sleep a night. Getting too much sleep, researchers have found, can be nearly as bad as getting too little. While exact requirements vary widely from person to person, you can surely find your "sweet spot" between that range, and you and your body will be all the better if you can stick to it every night.

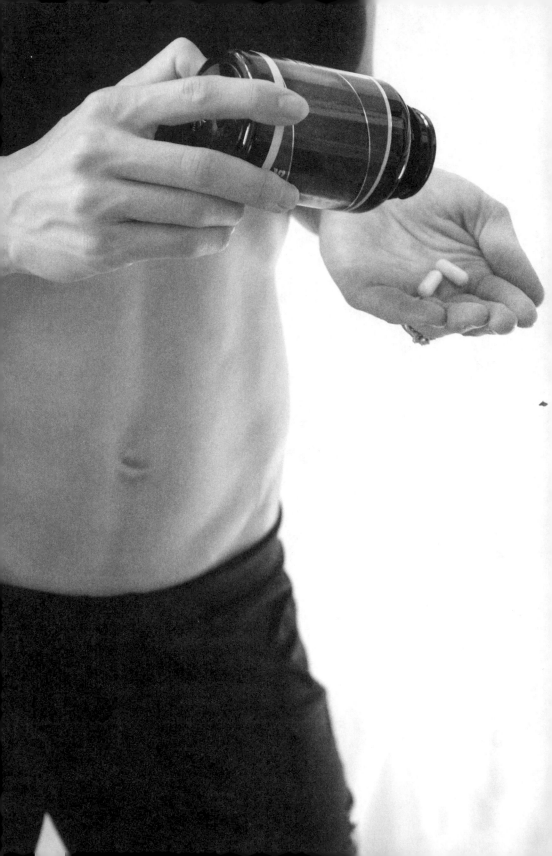

2

Nutrition: The Foundation for Everything

One of the most common things people say when they make up their minds to get in shape is, "I'm going on a diet." And most people fail. They set themselves up for failure by doing exactly what they said they were going to do: they went on a diet.

The term *diet* used to refer to a set of specific foods that people eat, but the meaning has been changed by popular culture and late-night infomercials. Now, a diet is generally considered to be a special meal plan someone is undertaking in order to lose weight. As such, diets are finite things. They have a set time to start, and at some point they end.

If your new diet has you eating right, working out regularly, and taking care of yourself with a particular goal in mind, you're going to see results. As long as you keep dieting, you'll continue to see results, and you'll feel great, live well, have more energy, and love what you see when you look in the mirror. But when the diet ends, the person you see in the mirror is going to look an awful lot like the person you saw when you started your diet to begin with. As soon as you return to your old eating habits, you'll regain all the weight that you lost—and probably even tack on a few extra pounds. For this reason, you can't succeed by dieting. You will always fail if you try because, at some point, your diet—by definition—has to end.

Diet vs. Lifestyle

Instead of going on a diet, I encourage you to adopt a new lifestyle that involves eating healthy. Nothing about getting in—and subsequently remaining in—good shape and good health can be temporary. Diets are temporary. You need to make consistent, healthy eating as much a part of your life as getting dressed every day. Make it a part of your life, day in and day out, and not something you start and end at a set time or date.

To understand the difference between a diet and a lifestyle, it helps to compare the dichotomy to a job versus a career. Most people—though not all—tend to look at jobs as placeholders, something to pay the bills before their ship comes in, so to speak. Maybe they're working at a fast-food restaurant while interviewing for a corporate position, or maybe they're working in a warehouse while finishing law school. Regardless, they don't put everything they've got into it because they're waiting for it to end. That isn't to say they hate their work, but it isn't their lifelong passion. They see it as effort.

A career, on the other hand, is something people put their heart and soul into. They roll with the punches, the ups and down, they're prepared to weather a storm or two (or five or ten) no matter what it takes. They're so engrossed in its success that it doesn't seem like effort. No matter the obstacles—the easy stuff and the harder stuff, the adjustments and the new experiences—they're building the brand, building the business, preparing to live on it for as long as possible.

A diet is a job. A lifestyle is a career.

I'm not trying to downplay the difficulty of dieting. It's hard. In fact, it's much harder than making a lifestyle change. Because when you decide to diet, you're convincing yourself that you're going to work extra hard—harder than ever, right? You're going to eat clean, avoid vices, and reach your goal. Whether that's to lose five pounds, fifteen pounds, or even fifty pounds, you're making a commitment to do whatever it takes to get there. And every step of the way, you'll be watching the mirror. You'll keep eyeing the scale. You'll keep pulling out the tape measure or that old pair of your favorite jeans you're just dying to fit back into. And each and every time you do this, you're wearing yourself down a little bit more. Little by little you're chipping away at the reserve of energy your mind put in place to get this diet over with. At some point, your resolve is going to break.

People justify a strict diet to themselves by saying, "Well, after I drop ten pounds, I can have a piece of cheesecake," or "Once I'm down to my goal weight, I can start having a couple of glasses of wine again." You restrict yourself from things you enjoy and desire, and you do it because you make them a reward for yourself after all the hard work. Unfortunately, those rewards are the very things that caused you to put on the extra weight in the first place.

The hardest part of changing the way you eat and starting to exercise is getting your mind in the right place to do it. Anyone can go through the motions of push-ups, sit-ups, squats, and lunges—and a thousand other movements—to get the heart rate up and burn a few calories. However, no one can burn enough calories through exercise to make up for a lifestyle of eating high-calorie, unhealthy foods in proportions that would otherwise feed a squad of junior high cheerleaders. So what's the answer? You don't diet. You change your lifestyle.

The Trickle-Down Effect of Making a Change

When you make a change to your lifestyle as a whole—when the very foundation of each day is based around feeling great and living longer so that you may enjoy your family, friends, and the things you love   the mental aspect becomes easy. There's no question about whether you can get through a diet or whether or not you can sacrifice such-and-such to reach your goal weight. You have now replaced thinking of food as a reward—like allowing yourself a dessert after every five pounds—with real benefits, like feeling more self-confident. You'll no longer say self-defeating things to yourself when you look in the mirror.

Now, a lot of people might be thinking: isn't that a lot to expect just from changing the way I eat and moving around a little more for exercise? Isn't food just a tiny part of life? How can it make that much difference?

The answer is: no, it isn't a lot to expect from changing such important aspects of your life. Food is a huge part of your life. It makes that much of a difference *and more.*

Food is one of the few things that we absolutely must have to survive. It's *what* we eat that makes all the difference. People say that eating well is easy. It's not. The more garbage that companies box up and put on shelves and call food—which seems to be increasing every day—the harder it is to find foods that are actually good for you. It's cheaper and cheaper for companies to make bad food that comes in boxes than it is to prepare, ship, and sell fresh foods.

Think of most supermarkets. Where is the fresh meat section? In the back. Where are the fresh fruits and vegetables? Off to the side. What do you have to walk past to get to them? Packaged noodles, frozen pizza, plastic-wrapped Twinkies, and sugar-filled pies. And let's be honest—because that's important when considering your health—those things can taste pretty good. So again, the only way to fight this problem is to change your lifestyle. You simply change the places you shop, and when you do have to go to the big-box stores, you don't browse the aisles full of packaged, sugary, and fat-laden foods because you know what you're there for—maybe milk, produce, or eggs that your meat market or farmers' market didn't have—and you're out in a flash.

Everything comes down to planning. By making the decision to eat well and exercise, you're fighting the status quo. A vast majority of people are overweight, and according to the Centers for Disease Control and Prevention (CDC) over one-third of American adults are *obese*, meaning they have a Body Mass Index over 30. Over 15 percent of children are also already obese. As of 2010, the CDC said not a single state in the country had an obesity rate of less than 20 percent. That means one in five people are obese. In 36 states, the rate is 25 percent or greater. That's one in four. In two of those states, it's 30 percent or more, meaning nearly one in three people are obese. So the fact that you're making up your mind to be healthier, to be more active, and to live better, you're going against the flow of traffic—and you should feel proud for doing so. But you can only get there by changing your lifestyle.

One thing is absolutely certain: you *can* do it!

Explaining Protein, Fats, Carbohydrates

The three types of nutrients that you're surely familiar with are protein, fats, and carbohydrates. At one time or another, each has been pinpointed as the biggest offender toward promoting obesity. The truth is that none of them are evil; as a matter of fact, they're all beneficial as long as you consume them in moderation.

Protein is a prime nutrient and is the building block of muscle. Protein is comprised of amino acids that are responsible for both repairing and creating new muscle tissue; it is also filling, leaving you feeling more satisfied after eating. Beef, chicken, and fish are good sources of protein.

Fats can be broken down to good and bad fats. Good fats can actually help you maintain a lean body composition and are a sustained source of fuel for physical activity. Bad fats, such as trans fats, not only add on unwanted pounds but also can raise your cholesterol, increase your blood pressure, and create a host of other cumulative side effects. Omega-3's, which are found in fish, are good fats. Bad fats include saturated fats, like what's in butter and cream.

Carbohydrates are the main source of fuel for the body as they are most easily burned. Sugars are the most common form of carbohydrates that, like fats, can be classified as good or bad. Simple sugars, like those found in soft drinks and candy, spike your insulin levels and promote fat storage. Slow-burning carbohydrates, such as those found in oats and whole grains, help balance your blood sugar and provide quality energy because they process slowly, allowing your insulin levels to stay relatively stable.

Fibers, Fruits, Vegetables

Everyone knows that fruits and vegetables are supposed to be healthy. One of the key reasons is because of the fiber that is contained within these foods. For most people, their knowledge of fiber is limited to knowing it's the stuff contained in Metamucil that makes you go to the bathroom. And while that's correct, that's not the entire truth behind the benefits contained in the two categories of fiber, which are soluble and insoluble. Each can offer you a host of benefits and should be a part of a well-rounded diet.

Soluble fiber can help lower blood cholesterol and lower your blood sugar. This is particularly beneficial if you are at risk for diabetes. You can find soluble fiber in foods such as fruits (citrus) and oats.

Insoluble fiber is the type that helps promotes processing in your digestive tract. This is what you'll find in wheat bran and many types of vegetables.

Water

Being dehydrated—meaning you're not taking in enough fluids—can cause a litany of problems in the body. Dehydration makes you feel fatigued, which means you'll feel like everything you do is more difficult. Even worse, it can cause the body to increase the feeling of hunger, which increases the likelihood that you'll overeat and take in excess calories. For these many other reasons, it's important to stay hydrated and drink plenty of water.

Everyone's requirement is different, but the old "eight glasses a day" is a good start. If you sweat during the day from training or working in a warm environment, you'll probably need more. The easiest way to make sure you're drinking enough is to simply have water everywhere you go. Take a water bottle. Sip constantly.

A note on coffee with your breakfast: people love having coffee right after they wake up. It tastes good, it helps wake you up, and it smells fantastic. But good things come to those who wait, right? If you're a coffee drinker, don't pour that cup of java until you've had at least 16 ounces of water. It will replace fluids lost during the night and it will help you more easily reach your goal of staying hydrated.

Goal-Oriented Foods

Certain foods and beverages pack a little extra punch, whether it's helping you burn more calories or making you feel better overall. Here's a quick look at a few categories you'll find beneficial and also interesting. Along with enjoying their perks, you can impress your friends with your knowledge.

Terrific Tea

Green tea is a great beverage. It contains antioxidants that help protect the body from diseases such as Alzheimer's and Parkinson's—and may even protect against certain forms of cancer—and it has a little bit of caffeine for a pick-me-up, but not quite as much as coffee. And along with helping boost the metabolism, it's calorie-free (so long as you don't add sugar).

Green tea isn't the only beneficial option in this class of beverage. Others, like black tea, fend off fat-promoting hormones. Cortisol, for example, is a stress hormone that, among other things, encourages belly fat. A study out of University College London found that drinking black tea can reduce levels of cortisol, helping you keep fat away from your middle.

The Benefits of Coffee

Have no fear, coffee is safe to drink. As a matter of fact, studies show that it is beneficial, depending on how you prepare it and how much of it you drink.

More and more we are seeing the results of studies that show coffee is vastly beneficial to the human body. Compared to those who don't drink coffee, coffee drinkers are at lower risk of type-2 diabetes, dementia, cancer, stroke, and Parkinson's disease. Not bad.

Coffee is the most commonly used source of antioxidants in the world, which helps prevent cell damage caused by free radicals. Additionally, the minerals in coffee help control blood glucose (blood sugar), which helps fight off diabetes.

It can't be all good, right?

Well, right. Coffee does contain caffeine (unless you go for the decaf, of course). And caffeine can raise your blood pressure or, if you drink it too late at night, prevent you from getting a good night's sleep. So the key here is moderation and timing your coffee consumption properly. Further, if you're pregnant, it's best to avoid more than moderate doses of caffeine entirely.

When I talk about coffee, realize that I'm talking about your standard black coffee. Not a venti-nonfat-organic-chocolate-frappuccino served with extra-hot-foam-low-whip-and-double-blended. I just mean coffee the way your parents or grandparents drank it. When you move beyond brewed drip coffee, you're buying a dessert, not a coffee. A Starbucks venti iced Java Chip, for instance, has 580 calories and almost 90 grams of sugar. Likewise, a venti white chocolate mocha—one of America's favorite beverages—has just as many calories and 75 grams of sugar. So differentiate: coffee is good. Dessert in a cup, not so good.

Metabolism and Energy-Boosting Foods

Hot peppers contain *capsaicin*, which has been shown to not only burn extra calories while you're doing nothing but also to help blunt hunger, thus reducing the amount you eat.

An apple a day keeps the doctor away—you've heard that one, right? The relationship between you and your doctor may or may not change based on your apple consumption, but by eating them you are indeed promoting good health. Along with being a quality carbohydrate, apples contain antioxidants that have been shown to boost endurance and strength. And when you can train longer and stronger, you're in a better position to burn fat and feel great.

Immunity and General Health-Boosting Foods

Dark chocolate is full of antioxidants and can also lower your blood pressure and, studies have found, even prevent heart attack and stroke—how about that for not feeling guilty next time you enjoy a square of the good stuff? Look for dark chocolate that is at least 70 percent cocoa, and stick with just one or two squares per day.

Yogurt is another favorite. Look for the words *live active cultures* on the container. These are healthy bacteria that keep your insides healthy and balanced.

Garlic, too, has been shown to contain an active ingredient (allicin) that fights infection and bad bacteria. Some studies have even shown people who regularly consume garlic catch fewer colds and have lower rates of some cancers compared to people who don't eat garlic.

Joint Relief Foods

The *Journal of Biological Chemistry* found that the spice *turmeric* can be used as an anti-inflammatory drug in a similar fashion as aspirin. Pineapple, too, contains an anti-inflammatory element called bromelain, which has also been likened in effectiveness to pharmaceutical drugs.

Similarly, seafood such as shrimp and salmon can help keep you moving smoothly. Shrimp is high in glucosamine and salmon is high in omega-3 fatty acids, which help support not just healthy joints but heart health, too.

Who knew that eating well has so many benefits? Well, now *you* do!

Destroying Food Myths

Plenty of myths revolve around the foods we all eat. So to help educate you and make you feel better about your choices going forward, it's time to crush a variety of nutrition myths.

Myth #1: Frozen vegetables are less nutritious than fresh. This all depends on what they're compared to, but it's likely frozen vegetables have the same amount of vitamins and nutrients than the fresh stuff you can buy at the grocery store. The reason is that fruits and vegetables start losing their vitamins as soon as they're picked. Frozen vegetables tend to be frozen within hours of being picked, whereas your local supermarket is likely to sell produce that, while considered fresh, may have taken a week or more to get there. The exception to this? If you can buy from a farmers' market or other venue where you're buying things picked that day or very, very recently.

Myth #2: There are negative-calorie foods. A negative-calorie food is one that would require more calories to digest than it contains. Celery in particular has been labeled a negative-calorie food. This is not the case. There are no negative-calorie foods.

Myth #3: Sports drinks are better than water when you're in training. You can't go anywhere that people work out without seeing plenty of colorful sports drinks. The marketing works extremely well: you work out, you sweat, you need a sports drink. But this is false. Unless you're working out in extreme heat or for long periods of time, water is the best way to replace your lost fluids. The majority of sports drinks have a great deal of sugar, which is meant to replace the glucose in your muscles. The problem is that the majority of the training population doesn't work out hard enough or long enough for this to be a necessity. As an alternative, you can get sugar-free sports drinks, but then you are ingesting artificial sweeteners.

Even if you don't have a problem with Sucralose or aspartame, your body tends to not need what's in the marketed beverages, so if nothing else, you're wasting your money.

Reading Food Labels

While I always advocate that you buy fresh food whenever possible, it's hard to argue with the convenience of packaged food. If you do buy packaged food, you should pay close attention to the information on the nutrition panel, often located on the side or back of the package. On the other hand, many of the claims made on the front of the package are meaningless.

The Nutrition Panel

For good measure, I take you through a nutrition label from top to bottom so you can see a real-life example of what you're being told in this tiny box:

PRODUCT: StarKist Chunk Light Tuna (2.6oz/74g pouch)

Nutrition Facts

Serv. Size: 1 pouch

The serving size tells you how many expected servings are in the entire package. In this case, the package constitutes a single serving; however, many packages contain two or more servings. When there is more than one serving in a package, the nutrition panel lists information for the serving size rather than the entire package.

Calories: 80   **Calories from Fat:** 5

This represents the calories *per serving* of the food contained inside and how many are from dietary fat.

Total Fat: 0.5g/1%

The grams amount is the total grams per serving. The percentage is based on a 2,000-calorie diet. Most people don't eat 2,000 calories a day, so this number is generally of little value to you.

> Saturated Fat 0g
>
> Trans Fat 0g

Polyunsaturated Fat 0g

Monounsaturated Fat 0g

The nutrition panel sometimes breaks down the quantity of different types of fats. Pay close attention to the saturated and trans fat amounts; you want to avoid high levels of these types of fat.

Cholesterol: 35mg/12%

Though high levels of cholesterol can be a serious health risk, more evidence is showing us that dietary intake of cholesterol does not have much of an affect at all on your risk for coronary disease.

Sodium: 300mg/13%

This is the amount of salt you're taking in. High levels of sodium can cause hypertension and other serious side effects, so try and keep this number under control. There's no definitive number that is "safe" for everyone, but generally, less is best.

Potassium: 220mg/6%

Potassium can help lower your risk of hypertension. While deficiency is very rare in the modern world, it is still an important nutrient found in fruits, vegetables, fish, and meat.

Total Carbohydrate: 1g / 0%

Dietary Fiber 1g / 4%

This breakdown offers you information on where your carbohydrates are coming from. If the total carbohydrate number is high, but the dietary fiber content is low, you're potentially looking at a high sugar content and should try and avoid this food.

Protein: 18g/32%

Here is where you'll find how much muscle-building power your food is packing. In general, if a food has 1gram of protein per 10 calories, you're looking at a quality food. In the case of tuna, you're vastly exceeding that, which is great.

Ingredients: Light tuna, water, vegetable broth, salt.

The nutrition panel always lists ingredients in the order that they're included in the product. Tuna is the first ingredient, which means that tuna makes up the largest single ingredient.

Although tuna doesn't contain any sugar, many packaged foods do. A good rule of thumb is to avoid buying any food that has sugar (or some form of sugar, such as cane syrup or high-fructose corn syrup) as one of the first three ingredients.

Front-of-Label Claims

You've probably noticed the many health benefits proclaimed on the front of food packages. Many of those claims and terms sound a lot better for you than they really are.

Sucralose and Aspartame: Artificial sweeteners have been bringing the taste of cola to the dieting masses for decades. But more and more research shows that the brain doesn't really distinguish the diet stuff from the regular. In fact, research suggests that the sweet taste of these drinks causes the body to release insulin, which promotes fat storage. Further, artificial sweeteners appear to hinder regulation of calorie intake, making people feel hungrier.

Multigrain: Although any food description with the term *grain* in it sounds really healthy, the fact is that slapping *multigrain* on a label is often a form of deceptive marketing. Multigrain really just means it's made from multiple grains. This is the same with terms like *12-grain*. Yes, maybe it's multigrain or maybe it's made with 12 different grains, but unless the label specifically says "whole grains," it's probably made with refined grains, which aren't as healthy for you as whole grains.

Made with whole wheat: This is another line that's meant to look good at first glance, but *made with* doesn't say how much. The food might be made with only a small percentage of whole wheat.

Natural and 100% Natural: Both of these terms insinuate something that may not be true. These terms make people think they're getting a pure food with nothing artificial, but because the Food and Drug Administration doesn't have any specific requirements for the word *natural*, there's no stopping manufacturers from including additives. When it comes to meat, it's worth noting that animals that have been treated with antibiotics and hormones can still have their product labeled as natural.

Organic: One of the most hot-button issues in the food industry revolves around the term *organic*. With legal definitions varying widely, you're often buying more expensive foods that still can contain non-organic ingredients (in general, "organic" labeling only requires 70 percent organic content). On packaged foods, look for labels that say "100% Organic" or at least, "USDA Organic," which must be at least 95 percent organic content.

So in general, what's the rule: to go organic or not?

Some studies have shown that organic milk contains significantly more omega-3 fatty acids than other milks. So when it comes to dairy, it may be worth the premium. The same goes for produce since fruits and vegetables are more susceptible to pesticides and their residues can end up in what you're eating.

Lastly, beef has been shown to carry over drugs such as clenbuterol, all the way to human bodies after consumption. So when it comes to meat, go organic whenever possible.

Another option when buying fruit and vegetables is to look for descriptions of how the food was grown. For example, if you don't want to risk ingesting the harmful chemicals in insecticides and pesticides, which can breach the outer layers and skin of things like cabbage, lettuce, and apples, shop for produce that's grown "without pesticides."

Sea salt: If you're trading table salt for sea salt, do it for flavor, not the supposed health benefits of the trace minerals sea salt may provide. There aren't enough trace minerals to make it worth the switch, and both the sea and table versions are equal in sodium.

Boosts Immunity (or Supports … or Maintains …): These are terms you'll find on the front of boxes or in fancy script outside of the ingredient list. Ignore all of these claims. Most of the time they have an asterisk that will—in very, very small font—tell you that their claims haven't been verified. And for those who say they have studies to support their claims, you should be very curious as to who funded the study.

Gluten-free: More and more often these days labels on products proclaim that they are gluten-free. Gluten is a protein that exists in wheat and other carbohydrates, and some people have problems with its digestion. People have varying degrees of sensitivity to gluten, the most severe being Celiac disease, which is an abnormal immune response to gluten. But even if you don't have Celiac disease, it doesn't mean gluten doesn't negatively affect you.

Without trying to diagnose a serious health issue in these pages, there are a few steps you can take to find out if you have an allergy or sensitivity to gluten. Abdominal distension or bloating, fatigue, and gas can occur in people who have issues with gluten. If you have these symptoms after eating foods containing wheat and other such products, you may want to try eliminating gluten for a period of time and see if the symptoms ease.

Let's say you feel fine after eating gluten, but you're the type of person who looks in the mirror and thinks you look a little "round." This could be from water retention that is—you guessed it—caused by gluten. Many people are just sensitive enough to gluten that they retain fluid and always feel a little bloated. Try a gluten-free meal plan for a while and see if you find it beneficial; it certainly can't hurt and if nothing else, you'll learn about your body.

How to Clean Up Your Cupboards

Here's an easy exercise. Go through your cupboards and throw away anything that includes the following ingredients:

- Hydrogenated oil
- Partially hydrogenated oil
- High-fructose corn syrup
- Modified food starch

The first two items are trans fats, which are entirely foreign to the body; the third is a highly processed sweetener that has zero nutritional value (as in, not coupled with nutrients as you'd find with the plain fructose of an apple); and the last is frighteningly vague. In the latter, the word *modified* isn't required to be explained. What happened to your food starch? Only the manufacturer knows. Because these foods are foreign to the body, they are difficult to process and encourage fat storage, and thus, weight gain.

Your New Nutrition Program

Knowledge is power, and you now have plenty of knowledge when it comes to making wise choices about what's fueling your body. Next it's time to learn how much you need.

Finding Your Body's Caloric Needs

The easiest method to find the appropriate caloric intake for your body is to track what you tend to eat and work backward or forward. The reason for this is that everyone's metabolism is different. For people who want to lose body fat, you need to reduce your caloric intake. For people who want to gain lean mass, you need to add calories.

Without changing your regular habits, write down everything you eat for three full days. Don't forget to include drinks—you may be taking in quite a few calories through various sugary liquids or alcohol. You can calculate your consumption with websites like www.caloriecount.com or www.calorieking.com or use the food log at the end of this chapter.

Once you have your three-day total, divide this number by three. This is your base consumption.

Calories for Fat Loss

If you're training to lose fat, you need to reduce your daily caloric intake. If you regularly consume 3,300 calories per day, try cutting back to 3,100 calories per day for a week and see how you feel. Reduce further if necessary, and when you find a calorie level that gives you the right balance of fat loss, energy, and strength, strive to maintain it.

When reducing calories, you may find it easier to eat several smaller meals a day. Often, when you reduce intake of calories, you'll be dealing more often with hunger. By eating frequently, you should be able to stave off any hunger pangs that might cause you to overeat.

Calories for Muscle

If you're not adding the amount of lean muscle you want, you're probably either not getting enough calories or not getting enough of the right kind of calories. But if you're not adding weight at all—meaning not gaining fat or muscle—then go ahead and adjust your caloric intake.

When looking to put on muscle, you need carbohydrates for fuel and protein for growth. Choose foods that, at the end of the day, will give you about 40 percent of your calories from protein, 30 percent from carbohydrates, and 30 percent from fats when you add everything up after your last meal of the day.

If you're looking to put on new muscle, try adding calories little by little, such as 200 at a time (a bit more than a can of tuna in water) each day for a week. If you still don't put on any new weight, you can add 200 more until you find the right calorie count for you.

You can include additional calories easily by eating more often throughout the day; Instead of three meals, eat five meals, and add a bit more food to one particular meal each time you need to up your calories.

Eat This, Not That

Snacking or, as it's sometimes called, "grazing" is responsible for a large number of calories that people eat. Often they don't even realize they're doing it, or recognize how a few bites here and a few bites there eventually add up to a lot of extra pounds on the hips. Part of that issue is also that people pick the wrong things to snack on or to make their meals with, and something that could generally be healthy, turns out to be calorie-heavy or sugar-laden. An easy fix is to simply substitute foods you used to eat or want to eat with other foods that are equally as tasty, but substantially better for you.

Here is a short list of just a few of the easy changes you can make as well as some things you can substitute in other meals/recipes:

Instead of ...	Try ...
Bacon	Turkey bacon
Processed Peanut Butter	All-Natural Peanut Butter
Soda	Sugar-free tea
Candy	Almonds
Cheese	Fat-free cheese
Regular salad dressing	Low-fat dressing/Fat-free dressing
White rice	Brown rice
White bread	Whole-grain bread
Sugar cereal	Oatmeal or granola
Butter	Applesauce (often able to use in place)
All-purpose flour	Whole-wheat flour (for half of the called-for amount)
Mayonnaise	Mayonnaise made with Olive Oil
Pasta	Whole-wheat pasta
Ice cream	Plain yogurt with fresh fruit
Guacamole	Salsa

Fighting Cravings

Everyone gets cravings. For some people it's chocolate, for others it is ice cream, wine, chips, or any variety of salty or sugary snacks. Indulging in a craving isn't the end of the world, but overindulging will definitely put you off course and take you away from your goals of getting lean and healthy. You have to learn to fight the cravings off and keep your mind focused on what you're trying to achieve.

The mental aspect really is the biggest obstacle to getting in shape. People become complacent with their bodies, their health, and their energy levels. Changing such attitudes is difficult because it takes breaking a habit. And on any level, changing a behavior that you've done for years or even decades is very challenging. But you can do it.

First, acknowledge you're having a craving. It's fine! They happen. But recognize it for what it is, think about when you last ate and when you realize that your body is only after junk that you don't need right now, get stern with yourself. Tell yourself it isn't going to happen, you're not going to go hunting down some food you don't need. Even ask yourself: *What good is this for me in the long run?* Ten minutes after you've eaten, you largely forget the flavors you just experienced. So why risk putting your progress back several days (if you take in an exponential number of calories in a splurge) for ten minutes of satisfaction?

Along with being mentally tough, you can also use these few tricks to make the cravings bite the dust:

Exercise

To push back cravings you don't have to start training for a marathon, you need only do something as simple as go for a walk to get the same satisfaction. Surprising, but true! Sweets cause the body to release endorphins, which make you feel good. Exercise does the exact same thing. And when you fight a craving with exercise, you're doing double-duty for improving your body.

Distract Yourself

Make a list of things you need to get done around the house, work you haven't had time for, or little errands that aren't priorities but still need to be taken care of. Then, whenever you find yourself just combing the cupboards for a snack, take to the list instead. You'll feel more satisfied that you're getting things done *and* you'll be avoiding calories you didn't need in the first place.

Give It a Rest

Lack of sleep puts a lot of strain on your body, which it tries to make up for by taking in excessive amounts of calories. If you find yourself hungry but also tired, try taking a short nap. You'll likely be surprised at how beneficial it is for your waistline if you start catching up on sleep.

Drink Water

Dehydration can cause you to feel hungry even when you're not in need of any food. If you're fighting a craving, try drinking a glass or two over 15 minutes or so and see if it has passed.

Chew Gum

Sugar cravings are often the worst kind to fight, but you can often keep them at bay simply by chewing some sugarless gum. The sweet flavor satisfies the mind's desire and helps you keep off the pounds.

The Costs of Healthy Eating

One of the most common arguments against eating healthy is that it is cost prohibitive. Time and time again people fall back on the excuse that they simply cannot afford to eat better. The phrase, "It's cheaper to eat McDonald's than it is to eat healthy," is one that has been uttered over and over. And it's a lie.

Here's a cost breakdown of some popular food choices and some healthy options in contrast. The results will surprise you.

	McDonald's Extra Value Meals	*Tuna Fish Sandwich*
Price:	$5.39 to $7.29	$4.07 ($.59 for one can tuna fish; $1.49 for a loaf of 100% whole-wheat bread), $1.99 mayo with olive oil
Serves:	1	1 (with lots of bread and mayonnaise left over!)
	Large three-topping take-out pizza	*Grilled chicken and brown rice*
Price:	$10	$3.28 (1 lb. chicken breast $1.89; 1 lb. brown rice $1.39)
Serves:	4	4
	Cheeseburger and fries from sit-down chain restaurant	*Homemade lean hamburger and baked fries*
Price:	$8.99	$8.96 (1 lb. lean ground beef, $3.49; 5-lb. bag of potatoes, $1.99; 1 lb. tomato, .99 cents; One package low-fat cheese slices, $2.49)
Serves:	1	4

Note: All prices were taken from Seattle-area restaurants and supermarkets in March 2012.

Additionally, you can add fruits and vegetables to any of the meals in the right column for a nominal cost and still be well under the "fast food" option costs, and be significantly healthier, to boot.

As I hope these comparisons prove, you can eat more cheaply and healthfully at home. So what excuses do you have left? You could, of course, use the line, "I just don't like healthy food."

Well here's a shopping list of healthy foods—and odds are, you're a fan of plenty of them.

Shopping List

Protein sources:

> Bison
>
> Chicken breast
>
> Cottage cheese
>
> Crab
>
> Flank steak
>
> Lean ground beef
>
> Lean ground turkey
>
> Lean ham
>
> Lean roast beef
>
> Low-fat cheese
>
> Low-fat milk
>
> Low-fat yogurt
>
> Pork tenderloin
>
> Salmon
>
> Shrimp
>
> Tilapia
>
> Tri-tip steak
>
> Turkey breast

Grain carbohydrates:

> Brown rice
>
> Oatmeal
>
> Quinoa
>
> Whole-grain cereals (Quaker Oat Squares, Kashi, Cheerios)

Whole-wheat bagels

Whole-wheat bread

Whole-wheat English muffins

Whole-wheat pasta

Whole-wheat pitas

Whole-wheat tortillas

Vegetables:

Asparagus

Bell peppers

Broccoli

Cauliflower

Cucumbers

Onion

Romaine lettuce

Spinach

Sweet potatoes

Tomatoes

Fruits:

Apples

Bananas

Blueberries

Cherries

Oranges

Peaches

Strawberries

Timing Is Everything

So you know your calorie base and you have lots of good foods to choose from. Next, you need to know when you should eat what.

The body works in a very cyclical manner based on when you eat and when you sleep. Body processes, such as metabolism, slow down while you're sleeping and the body facilitates muscle repair and growth. It's important, then, to satisfy the needs of the body with a proper meal before bed. Similarly, the body will be in a fasted state when you wake up, and will be in great need of, among various things, amino acids and carbohydrates for energy and subsequent fuel.

But keep in mind that your body and your schedule are unique to you. "Breakfast" is a common term for the first meal, so I'm going to use that, but the rest are labeled more as what they are, and not the traditional "Lunch" and "Dinner." While these are terms that will never go away, they really aren't something you should focus on very much. "Lunch" is often looked at as "Noon," but if you're eating more often—as you should be— you may eat at 10:30 A.M. and not again until 1:30 P.M.; neither are lunch, just great meals to help keep you fueled for the rest of your day.

Breakfast

After you sleep—whenever that is—you're going to wake up at least somewhat dehydrated. Your body uses up water for respiration and other processes while you are asleep, so the first thing you need to do is drink water.

Your body is primed for burning fat after you wake up due to an absence of insulin-spiking foods while you slept, so keep that momentum by avoiding carbohydrates as much as possible. Stick with protein sources such as eggs.

Eggs are one of the most perfect foods known to man, full of protein and, given what they provide, relatively low in calories. Research also tells us that people who eat eggs for breakfast eat fewer calories throughout the rest of the day and ultimately burn more body fat.

Pre-Workout Meals

If you train in the middle of the day, try to eat at least two meals that contain carbohydrates before your workout. This is also a caveat to my previous suggestion that you avoid morning carbs: if you train shortly after waking, you'll want carbs in your first meal.

Post-Workout Meals

Unless you train at the very end of the day, make sure your post-workout meal also contains carbohydrates because you want a well-rounded balance of nutrition to take advantage of this post-workout window of recovery, where the body is better able to take up more of the nutrients you consume.

Last Meal of the Day

When possible, avoid carbohydrates in the last meal to prevent a spike of insulin, which will promote fat storage of unused energy (calories) that you'll still have when you go to sleep.

Your Personal Food Log

Making a food log might at first seem like a trivial exercise, but there's no better way to determine exactly why your body composition is the way it is than looking at the exact foods you eat.

Keep track of your food intake for three days and then analyze your results. Here is how it works:

Food/Drink: Write down whatever you eat or drink and in what quantity.

Calories: If you don't have this information from the package or menu, you can fill in this section later by using online tools such as caloriecount.com.

Time: Keep track of the time of day each time you consume something. This is great information to have to determine if you go long periods of time without food, or if you graze all day long. It's also good to determine whether or not you're eating a lot of sugary foods right before bed.

Day 1

FOOD/DRINK & AMOUNT	CALORIES	TIME

Day 1 Total Calories: _____

Day 2

FOOD/DRINK & AMOUNT	CALORIES	TIME

Day 2 Total Calories: _____

Day 3

FOOD/DRINK & AMOUNT	CALORIES	TIME

Day 3 Total Calories: _____

Day 4

FOOD/DRINK & AMOUNT	CALORIES	TIME

Day 4 Total Calories: _____

Day 5

FOOD/DRINK & AMOUNT	CALORIES	TIME

Day 5 Total Calories: _____

Day 6

FOOD/DRINK & AMOUNT	CALORIES	TIME

Day 6 Total Calories: _____

Day 7

FOOD/DRINK & AMOUNT	CALORIES	TIME

Day 7 Total Calories: _____

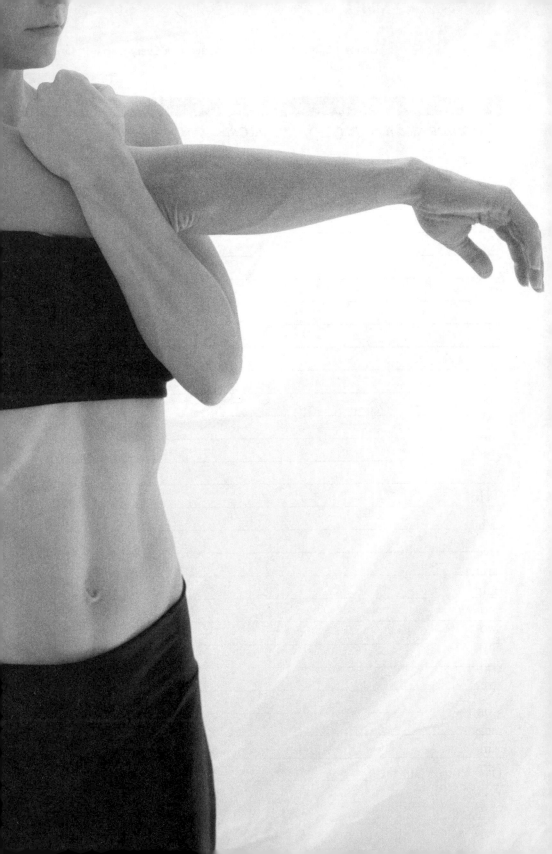

3

Stretching Out

Stretching is by and large a very simple thing. You probably do it all the time and don't even think about it: when you get out of bed and raise your arms to loosen up, when you get out of the car and twist your neck and back after a long drive, or maybe even when you're sitting and reading this book and straightening your legs. But there are proper ways to stretch and risky ways to stretch, and in this chapter I teach you the difference and show you ways to loosen up your entire body.

The Basics of Stretching

Why stretch?

Over the last couple of years, people have become a bit disenchanted with stretching because some studies indicate that stretching can reduce power output for a short period afterward, thus preventing maximal strength and muscle growth. Using these studies to justify not stretching presents two problems: first, you don't generally want to stretch before a workout, anyway; and second, you don't stretch to build or shape muscle. So the arguments against stretching are moot. To understand why you *should* stretch, keep reading.

Contrary to what many people say, stretching *is* exercise. Stretching puts tension on the muscle(s) involved and creates a muscular response. It's the same cause and effect that you get with a bench press or squat, but the difference is the end result. When you do squats, you're doing an exercise to create stronger, more muscular thighs. When you stretch, you're doing an exercise to elongate your muscles and increase your flexibility.

Stretching can be broken down into seven different types, but for our purposes, we need only focus on the two most basic types of stretches:

A *dynamic stretch* is one that involves active motion to stretch the muscles. A body-weight squat, for instance, could be considered a dynamic stretch (if done properly) because it lengthens the muscles of the leg. Arm swings and body twists are other examples of dynamic stretches. When you perform a series of dynamic stretches to prepare for an activity, you're doing an active warm-up.

A *static stretch* is a stretch in which you reach a position where the body can naturally go no further, and you hold that position. An example of a static stretch is when you bend at the waist to try to touch your toes.

Stretching Do's and Don'ts

Do make stretching a regular part of your day. It doesn't take more than 10 or 15 minutes to get a good session of stretching in, and the benefits are incalculable.

Don't do static stretching as a warm-up. This likely goes against everything you ever heard in gym class when you were a kid, but static stretching as a warm-up is not safe. Trying to lengthen a cold muscle is a recipe for disaster.

Do a warm-up before stretching. We cover the best way to do this next.

Don't "bounce" your stretches. Again, this is probably something that goes against the elementary school wisdom you learned years ago, but it's another safety hazard. You should lean further into a stretch if it's comfortable to do so, but never use momentum to push yourself into a position you weren't meant to reach.

Do dress for successful stretching. It only takes a few seconds to change from your jeans into a pair of shorts or sweats, so make sure you do that. Wearing the wrong clothing can prevent you from reaching your full potential when stretching.

Don't let it hurt. You should be able to feel your stretching, but it shouldn't be painful. If you experience discomfort beyond the release of a tight muscle, stop immediately.

How Often?

Stretching is something that you can do often and continue to get results from, but like anything, you can overdo it.

Try stretching at least 15 minutes every day. If you can't do it every day, shoot for at least four times a week. If you don't stretch for a few days in a row, your muscles can pretty quickly stiffen up again and you'll have to start anew. Don't let your hard work go to waste; keep up on it and keep reaping the benefits.

Safe Stretching

You already know that you shouldn't start stretching when you're "cold," such as right off the couch after watching a movie or immediately after getting out of bed in the morning. Instead, you should do some simple movements to prepare your body for lengthening its muscles. The time at which you do this is going to depend on whether or not you are working out that day.

If you're training on a given day, simply stretch after your workout when your body is warm and muscles are already prepared.

If you're not planning to train that day, do some basic movements such as arm swings, knee lifts, gentle squats, calf raises, and some easy push-ups before stretching.

Upper Body Stretches

Keeping your upper body loose and limber is particularly beneficial for any activities that involve reaching upward. Whether that's as simple as grabbing a coffee mug out of the cupboard or loading things onto shelves, you'll find things much easier if you keep your neck, arms, back, and chest stretched out.

Leaning Neck Stretch

Stand up tall and place your right arm behind you, keeping it straight. Bring your left arm behind your back and grab your right wrist, then lean the neck away from the extended arm as if you were trying to touch your ear to your shoulder. Repeat on the opposite side.

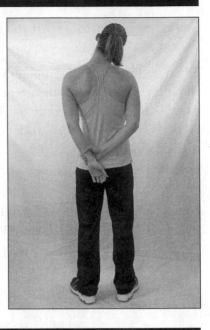

Chest Stretch on Wall

Stand facing a wall, extend your arm, and press your arm against the wall with your palm flat against the wall. Slowly turn your body away from your arm while maintaining contact with the wall with your hips and chest. Repeat on the other side.

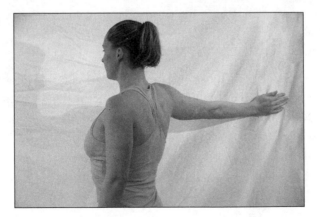

Chest Stretch on Wall 2

Stand facing a wall, place both arms on the wall above you, and step back so that your head can pass between your arms. Without moving your palms, slowly lean down until you feel a good stretch in your arms and chest.

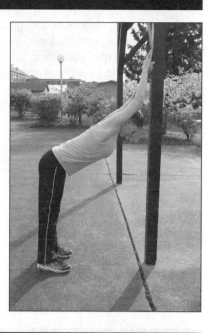

Biceps Stretch

Stand facing a wall and extend your arm so that the back of your hand is pressed against the wall. Slowly turn your body away from your arm while maintaining contact with the wall with your hips and chest. Repeat on the other side.

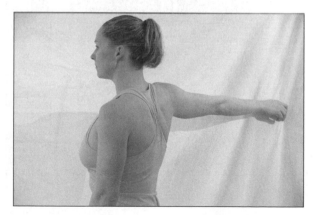

Raised Triceps Stretch

Sit or stand with your back straight and raise one arm straight up. Bend your arm at the elbow so that your hand is behind your head. Using your other arm, reach up and gently pull the raised elbow toward the opposite side. Repeat on the other side.

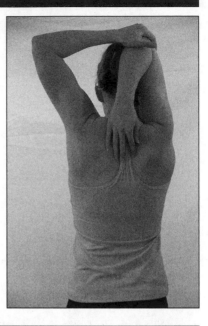

Cross Body Stretch

Standing up straight, cross one arm in front of your body and use the other arm to create a light stretch.

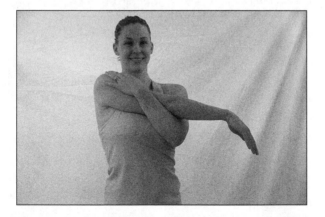

Towel Stretch

Take one end of a towel in your hand and place it behind your back, thumb facing upward. Take the other end of the towel in your other hand, thumb facing down, and draw it gently upward above your head until you feel your shoulder stretch.

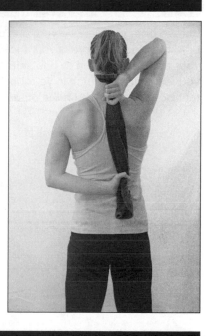

Lean Stretch

Sit down in a chair and lean forward a bit. Extend both arms forward, clasp one hand in the palm of the other, and roll your shoulder blades forward to get deeper into the stretch.

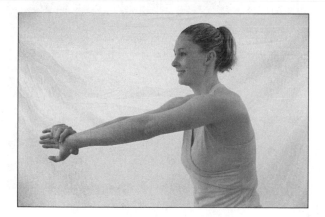

Streamline Stretch

Extend both arms above you, one overlapping the other, and press your biceps into your ears. Slowly lean to one side; when you feel a good stretch in your back, hold that position. Repeat on the other side.

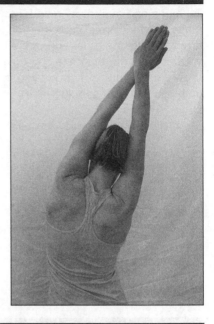

Forearm Stretch

Extend your fingers so your hands are flat. Place your fingers on the edge of a table, counter, or some other flat object, and push your palms forward.

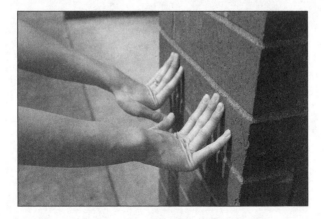

Forearm Stretch 2

Place your hands together in a prayer position and use your fingers on one hand to push back on your fingers on the other, holding at the stretched position. Alternate which side you push on.

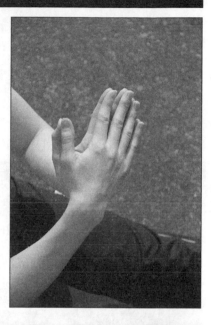

Seated Forearm Stretch

Sit on the floor and place your hands flat on the ground next to you. Slowly slide your hands behind you, keeping them completely in contact with the ground until you can't move them any further without lifting the palms.

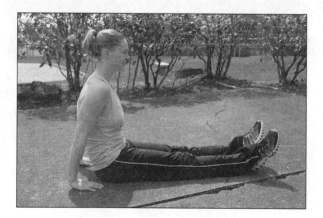

Core Stretches

Whether you have a job that involves a lot of sitting or a lot of standing, you've probably had to deal with pain in your lower back. Often, this has to do with a lack of flexibility in the lumbar. Once you loosen up your core, you'll find sitting or standing to be much more comfortable.

Abdominals and Obliques

Ab Lean

Lie on your stomach with your body lengthened out and slowly push your upper body toward the ceiling with your arms, leaving your legs in place. Push yourself back until you can feel your abdominals stretch.

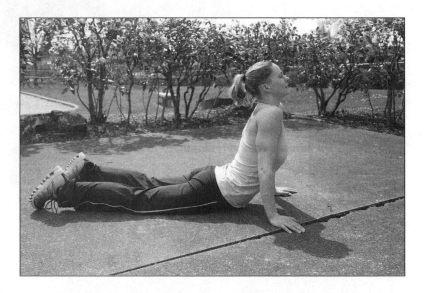

Lower Back and Hips

Hip Rotations

Stand up straight with your feet together and slowly lift one knee in front of you until your thigh is horizontal to the ground, then rotate your leg to the side as far as possible, and return your foot to where you started. Alternate with the opposite leg.

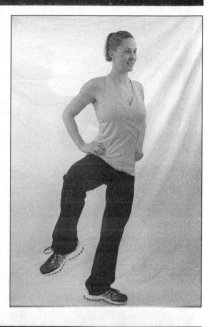

Hip Flexor Stretch

Move into a lunge position, with one knee on the ground and the other knee up with that leg's foot on the ground. Lean forward slightly until you feel a stretch in your hips and thigh.

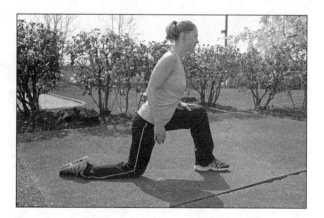

Twisting Hip Stretch

Sit on the ground with one leg extended and the other leg crossed over it. Bend at the knee until the crossing leg is positioned with the foot flat on the ground. Now rotate the body until your arms cross over the leg and use your arm to press against the bent leg, further rotating you and stretching the hip. Switch sides and repeat.

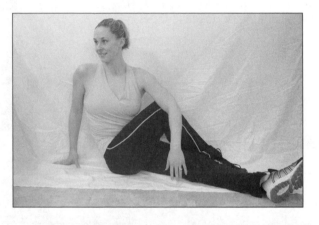

Butterfly Stretch

Sit on the floor and bend at the knees, allowing the knees to fall out to the sides, and pull the heel back until the bottoms of your feet touch. Hold your ankles with your hands and use your elbows to apply slight pressure inside the knees to push them toward the floor.

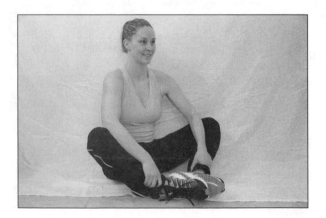

Inner Thigh Stretch

Stand with your feet a comfortable distance outside the shoulders. Place your hands on your hips and lean to one side until you feel a stretch on the inner portion of the thigh. Alternate legs.

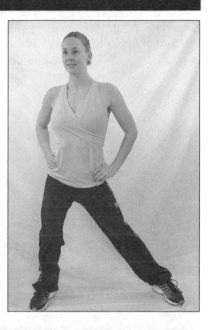

Lower Back Stretch

Lie on your back and draw the knees up toward the chest. Gripping behind the knees or around the legs with your arms, pull your knees upward gently.

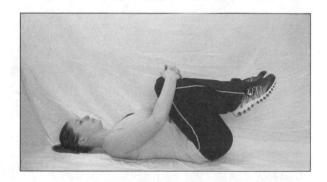

Hip Stretch

Sit on the ground with one leg in front of you and the knee bent, bottom of the foot pointing to the side. Place the other leg behind you and lean forward slowly.

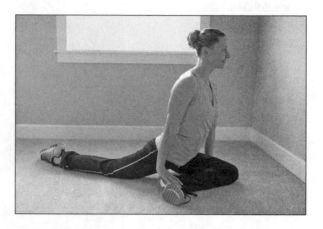

Groin Stretch

Sit on the floor with your legs straight and pointed out, making a V-shape with your legs. Extend your arms forward and lean as far as possible.

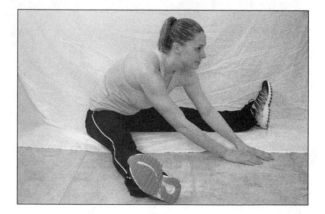

Seated Hip Stretch

Sit in a chair with a flat seat (one that doesn't dip) and draw one leg up, placing its ankle on top of the other leg. Use your hands to hold the bent leg steady, and lean forward to stretch.

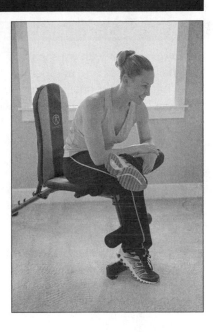

Lower Body Stretches

It seems like there's always a good amount of walking to be done, whether you're in the grocery store, at the mall, or parking a few blocks away from where you work. Then add the stairs—which you should take instead of the elevator—and you quickly realize how tight your legs can feel. These stretches will help make all of your walking (or running or jumping) much more comfortable.

Quadriceps

Standing Quadriceps Stretch

Stand up straight with your feet close together. Choose a leg and bend at the knee, bringing your heel toward your butt. Use your hands to steady the leg and pull it back toward you gently. Alternate legs.

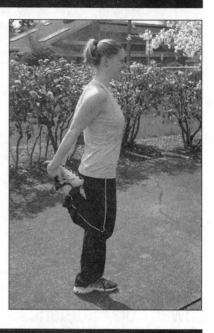

Seated Quadriceps Stretch

Sit on the floor with one leg straight out in front of you and the other bent with the heel just off to the side of your body. Lean back slowly over the foot behind you. Alternate legs.

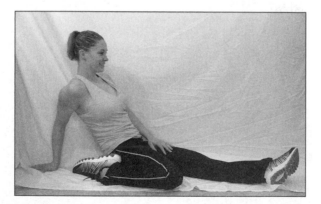

Facedown Quadriceps Stretch

Lie facedown on the ground with your legs straight and toes pointed. Bend the right heel up toward your butt and reach for the foot with your right hand and pull it closer until you feel the quad stretch. Repeat on the left side.

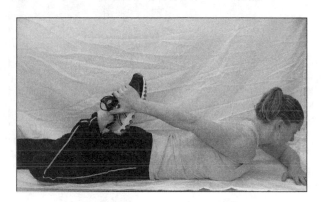

Hamstrings and Glutes

Hamstring Lean

Stand with your legs nearly straight and feet almost together. Lean forward and reach for your toes, stopping when you feel the stretch in your hamstrings. Be sure not to bounce your body to try and reach further.

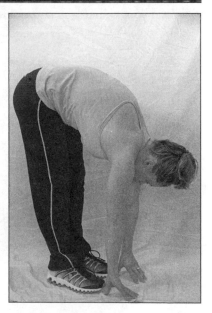

Knee Pull

Lie on your back with legs extended. Draw one knee up toward your chest and place your hands below your knee, pulling gently toward your head.

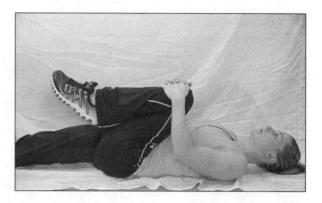

Seated Hamstring Stretch

Sit on the ground with your legs extended in front of you. Slowly lean forward and reach out with your arms toward your toes. Pause when you feel the stretch in your hamstrings and/or lower back.

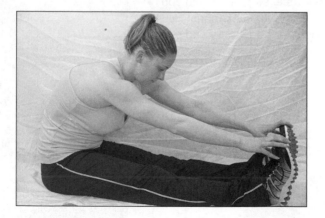

Cross-Leg Hamstring

From a standing position, cross one leg over the other and slowly lean forward, reaching for your toes as far as possible. Alternate legs.

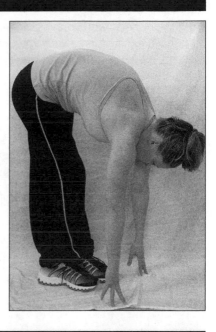

Elevated Hamstring Stretch

Place your heel on the seat of a chair. Keeping your standing leg nearly straight, lean toward your toes until you feel your hamstrings begin to stretch. Alternate legs.

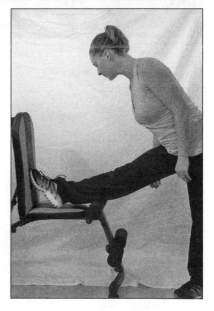

Lifted Hamstring Stretch

Lie on your back with your legs extended. Lift one leg up and, keeping it straight, bring it back toward your head, using your hands to keep the leg steady. Repeat with the opposite leg.

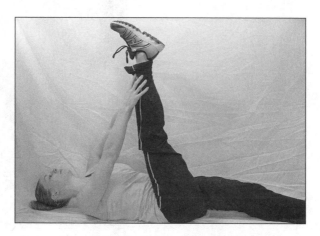

Calves

Wall Calf Stretch

Place the ball of your foot against the top of a baseboard or lower part of a wall and lean into it gently.

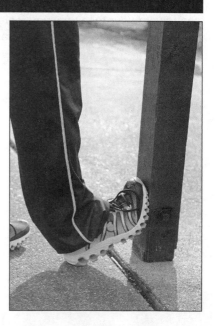

Wall Calf Stretch 2

Place your hands on a wall and your feet about a foot apart. Draw one leg back until the leg is nearly locked out and lean forward gently to stretch the calf of the back leg.

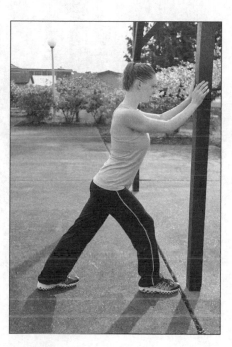

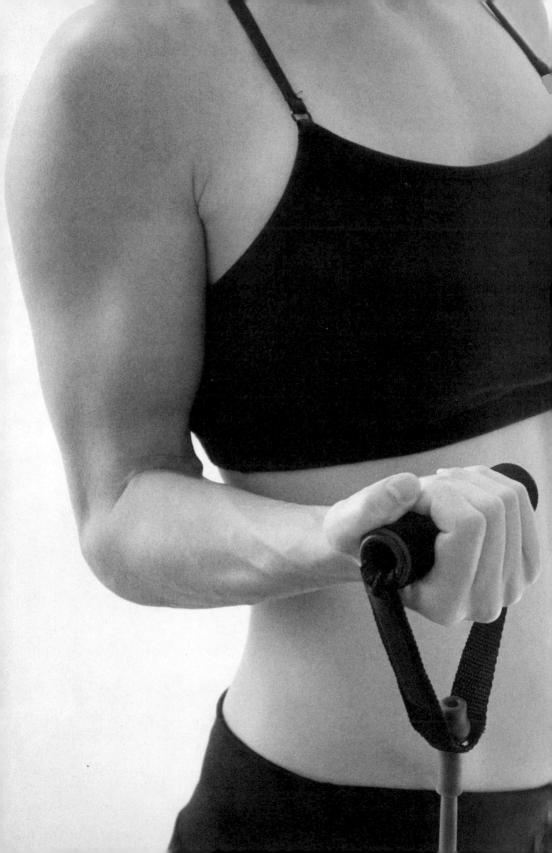

4

Upper Body Training

The muscles of the shoulders, chest, and arms are the first things people see when you catch their eye. They're also the muscles you first notice when you look at yourself in the mirror. Having well-defined muscles will surely increase your self-confidence and motivation for healthy living.

Arms

The common misconception about arm training is that to get really beautiful arms, you have to focus on curls and other movements that isolate the biceps. That just isn't the case! In fact, the triceps muscles—the back of your arm—makes up two-thirds of the size of your arms. To develop arms you're proud of and that leave an impression, make sure your arm training is well rounded.

Cable Curls

Stand on the center of a stretch-cord or resistance cable with the handles in your hands and your elbows at your sides. Keeping the elbows in place, curl your hands—fingers facing you—toward your chest.

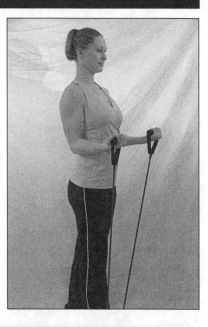

Cable Hammer Curls

Cable hammer curls are similar to cable curls, with the only difference being the position of your hands. In this exercise, position your hands so that your thumbs face toward the ceiling, and then curl your hands toward your chin.

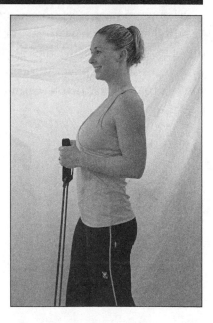

Triceps Dips

Find a solid object such as a bench or edge of a couch (remove the cushion), face away from it, and place your palms down on it with fingers wrapping over the edge. Extend your legs and move your body away from the object just enough so that you're balancing on your heels and can clear the object as you go down. Extend your arms so that you're holding yourself up, slowly lower yourself until your butt is just off the ground, and then return to the starting position.

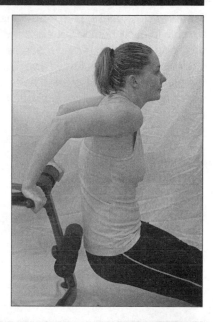

Triceps Cable Extensions

Stand with your legs slightly staggered and your feet just outside shoulder-width. Lean forward from the waist and bend your knees slightly. On the side of the leg that's forward, hold a portion of a cable close to your forward knee. With your other hand, grasp a handle of the cable and extend the arm backwards, keeping the elbow in close to the body.

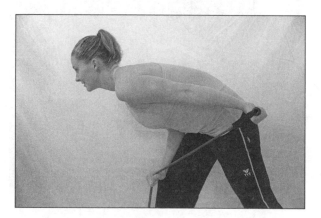

Overhead Extensions

Standing up straight, take a portion of a cable in hand behind your back. With your opposite hand, grasp a handle of the cable, raise your arm above you. Bend at the elbow and bring the hand behind your head, hold it, and then extend back to the top.

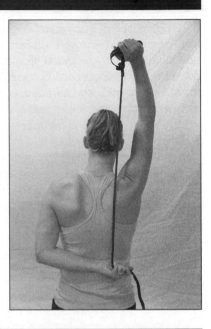

Triceps Push-Ups

Assume a standard push-up position (described later in this chapter) but bring your hands in closer so that they are aligned with your shoulders. Lower yourself down just as with a push-up until you're only a few inches off the ground, pause, and then return to the starting position.

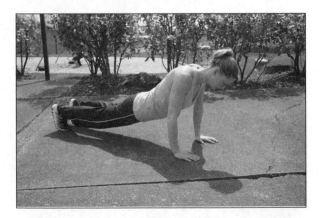

Medicine Ball Triceps Extensions

Stand up straight and raise a medicine ball above your head, holding it in both hands. Keeping your elbows next to your ears, bend from the elbow down and lower the medicine ball behind your head, pause, and then raise it back up.

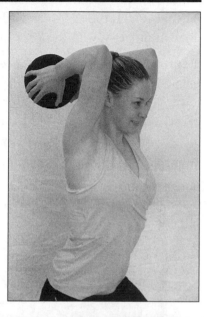

Medicine Ball Arm Curls

Take a medicine ball in one hand and keep your arm at your side. Curl your hand upward, and then slowly lower it back down. When your arm is extended downward, keep it slightly bent to keep tension on the muscle.

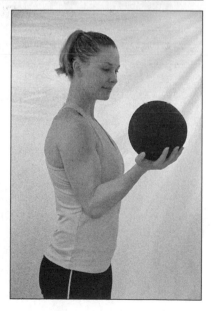

Chest

The push-up is the most standard of all chest exercises, though it's often done improperly, with the arms too close together.

To properly do a push-up, balance on the balls of your feet with your back flat and your arms extended, hands placed just outside the shoulders. Slowly lower yourself down until your chest is about four inches from the floor, pause, and push back up to the starting position. At no point do you want to lock your arms out, though; always maintain a slight bend.

You can increase the variety of this exercise by moving your hands farther out to the sides.

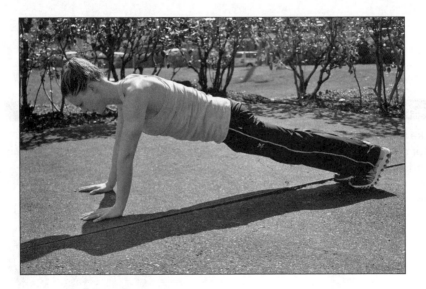

Incline Push-Ups

Find a solid object with a flat surface, such as a stair or heavy bench. Place your arms equal distances outside of your shoulders and balance on the balls of your feet. Slowly lower yourself toward the surface until your chest is a couple of inches away, pause, and then return to the starting position.

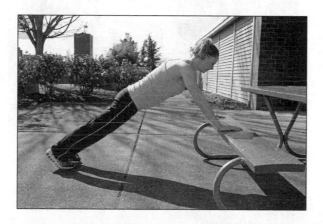

Decline Push-Ups

Find a solid, flat object where you can place the tops of your feet. Extend your body out and balance on your hands, which are placed just outside the shoulders on the ground. Ideally, you want your feet to be up on an object high enough that your back is horizontal to the ground. Slowly lower yourself until your chest is a few inches from the ground and then return to the starting position, making sure not to lock your elbows.

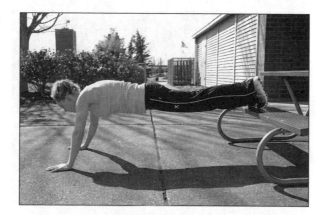

Exercise Ball Push-Ups

Balance yourself with your toes on an exercise ball and your hands on the floor. Keep your back straight and lower yourself down as with a traditional push-up.

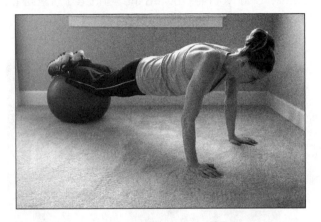

Alternating Leg Raise Push-Ups

These types of push-ups give you more practice keeping your entire body in alignment while you train.

This move starts in the traditional push-up position. The difference here is that, as you lower yourself down, you lift your left leg, returning it to the ground as you return to the starting position. Then, you repeat the maneuver with the right leg. After both legs, you have done *one* rep.

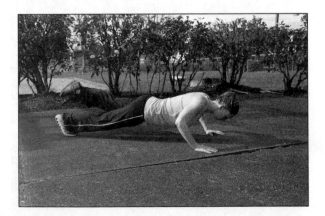

Dip Push-Ups

Take a push-up position but widen your arms an extra four to six inches. Instead of lowering yourself straight down, lower yourself toward one hand, pause a couple of inches above the ground, and then return to the starting position.

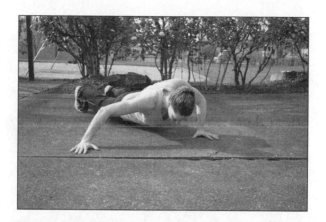

Plyometric Push-Ups

This is a more advanced push-up technique. Start in a traditional push-up position and lower yourself down. When you push to go upwards, instead of the slow and controlled movement of the standard variation, push yourself with force so that your hands leave the ground. As you land, keep the elbows bent to ensure a soft landing, and then go right into the next push-up.

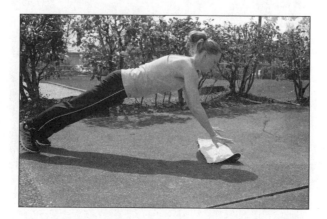

One-Hand Medicine Ball Push-Ups

Place one hand on a medicine ball and the other flat on the ground with the rest of your body in a traditional push-up position. Lower yourself slowly and pause a couple of inches from the ground, then push yourself back up. After each rep, switch hands by placing the floor hand on the exercise ball and moving the ball hand to the floor.

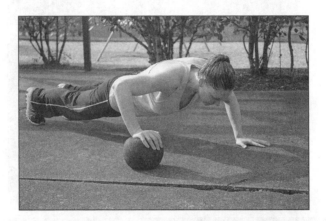

Two-Hand Medicine Ball Push-Ups

Place both hands on a medicine ball, keeping your core tight. Lower yourself down until your chest is just off of the ball, and then push yourself to the starting position.

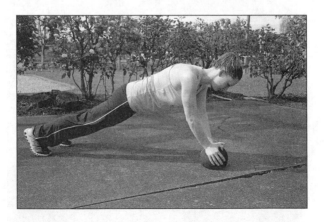

Cable Chest Presses

Place an exercise cable or resistance band around a post or column and face away from the post with a handle in each hand. Lift your elbows to the height of your shoulders and place your hands facing forward. Press your hands forward as if doing a push-up until the hands are nearly together, then slowly return to the starting position. For increased resistance, step farther away from the post.

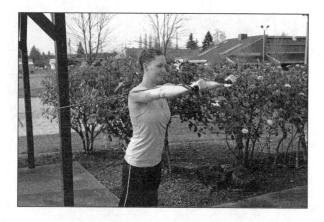

Cable Post Flies

Place an exercise cable around a column or post and face away from the post with a handle in each hand. Start with your arms straight out to your sides with only a slight bend at the elbows. Keeping the arms straight, pull the cable and bring the hands together in front of you. Pause at the contraction, and slowly return to the starting position.

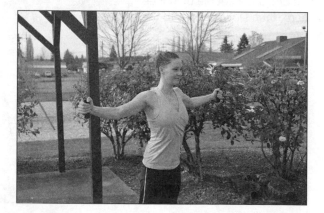

Shoulders

Shoulder Push-Ups

Put yourself in an inverted V by placing your hands on the ground while standing and moving your feet back just a foot or two. Slowly bend at the elbows to bring yourself closer to the ground, then push yourself back into the starting position.

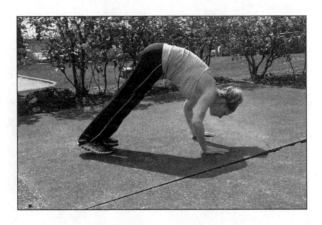

Cable Overhead Presses

Stand in the center of a cable and take the grips in hand. Keeping your elbows at your sides, bring your hands up to the side of your face, palms facing forward. Press both hands up evenly above your head until your hands are just a couple of inches apart. Pause here, then slowly return to the starting position.

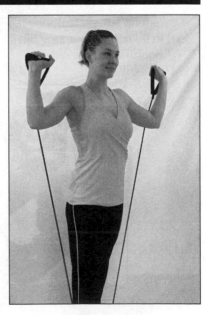

Side Laterals

Stand on a cable cord and take one handle into your hand, relaxing your arm at your side. Keeping a slight bend in the elbow, raise the arm out to your side, palm facing down, until the hand is just above the shoulder. Pause, and then slowly return to the start position.

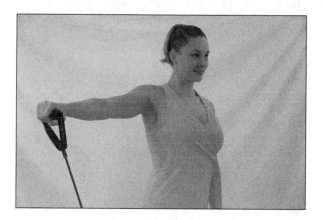

You can do this exercise with two arms a time.

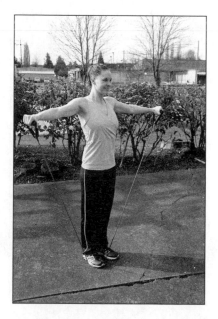

Front Laterals

Standing on a cord, one hand at your side, grip the handle so that your palm is facing behind you. Slowly raise your arm forward while maintaining a slight bend in the elbow. Pause when the hand is just above the shoulder, and then return to the starting position.

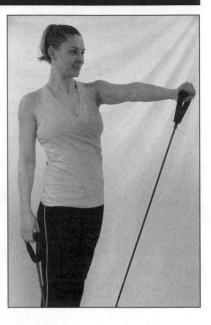

You can do this exercise with two arms at once.

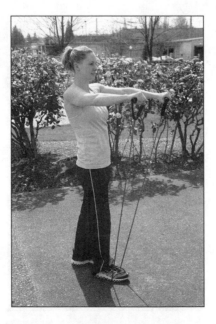

Rear Laterals

Stagger your feet and place a cable underneath your forward foot. Grip the handle with the arm on the opposite side of the forward leg and lean forward, keeping your back straight. With palm of the hand that's grasping the cable facing the side of your front leg, draw the arm out to your side, keeping the elbow slightly bent, until the arm is just higher than the shoulder. Pause, and then return to the starting position.

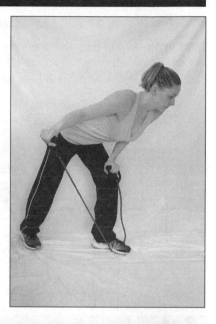

Hand Walks

Position yourself over the top of a sturdy couch back, facing behind the couch. Rest your thighs on top of the couch back and place your hands on the floor so that you are facing the floor. Now walk your hands down, moving the body to follow, from one side of the couch and back.

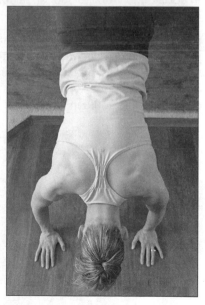

Walking Plank

You'll feel this exercise in your abs as well as your shoulders.

Start in a push-up position and then walk with your hands, slowing placing one in front of the other; walk yourself both forward and backward. Always keep a slight bend at the elbow and keep your back as flat as possible.

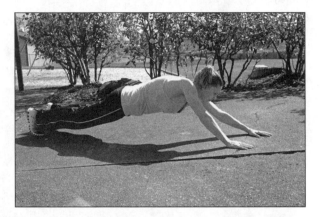

Diamond Push-Ups

In addition to working your shoulders, this exercise also works your triceps and chest.

Place your hands on the ground with your fingers and thumbs touching so that you're making a diamond shape with your thumbs and index fingers. Extend your body out into a push-up position, but keep your hands a bit further down below the chest than you would for a regular or triceps push-up. Lower yourself down as far as you can, and then push yourself back into the starting position.

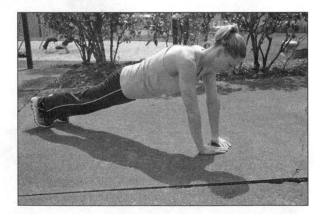

Medicine Ball Circles

Stand up straight with your knees slightly bent and hold a medicine ball in front of you with your arms extended. To start the movement, move your arms in a clockwise motion as if you're drawing a circle in the air and continue all the way around to the starting position. You can also reverse and make circles counter-clockwise.

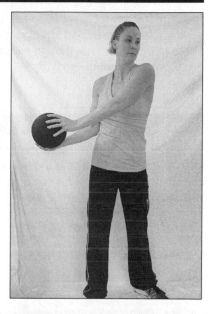

Overhead Medicine Ball Raises

Stand up straight and hold a medicine ball in your hands. Keeping your arms straight with just a slight bend, raise the ball above your head, pause there, and then lower it back down.

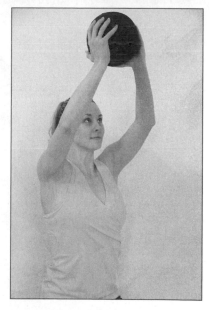

Back

A common term for great shape is having an "X" frame body. This involves having toned, developed shoulders, a trim waist, and defined, muscular legs. You can't get that look though without training your back. It isn't a glamorous body part, but exercising it is necessary and, fortunately, can be a lot of fun.

Exercise Ball Back Squeeze

Facing an exercise ball, balance by resting your hips on it. Extend your body slightly up at an angle and move your arms out to your sides. From here, squeeze your shoulder blades together, hold for three seconds, then return to the starting position and repeat.

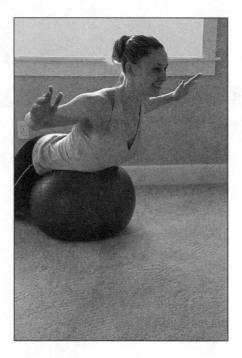

Table Pull

Lie underneath a table (or other solid object) and reach up and grip the edge. Maintaining a flat back, balance on your heels and pull yourself up as far as possible, pause, and then slowly return to the starting position.

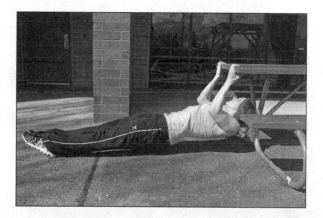

One-Hand Table Pull

Just as with the table pull, lie underneath a table (or other solid object). Using only one hand this time, grip the edge of the table. Cross the other arm over your body or grasp the pulling wrist for stability. Maintaining a flat back, balance yourself on your heels and pull yourself up as far as possible, pause, and then slowly return to the starting position.

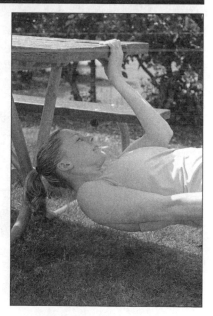

Lying Arm Raises: Front

Lie with your stomach on the ground and keep your toes pointed so that the tops of your feet are on the floor. Extend your arms out in front of you, palms facing down, and lift your chest. Then, touch your fingertips to the ground before lifting the arms as high as possible. Pause at the peak, then repeat.

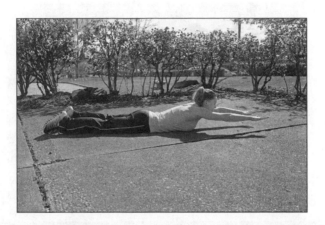

Lying Arm Raises: Side

This is similar to front raises except you extend your arms out to your sides. When lifting your hands off the ground, try and squeeze the shoulder blades together. Pause at the peak of contraction before lowering them back down.

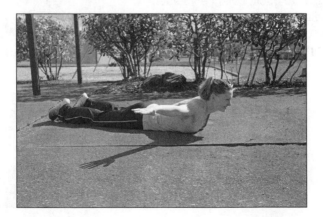

Medicine Ball Rows

Stand up with your knees slightly bent. Hold a medicine ball with both hands, lean forward, and extend your arms down, holding the medicine ball beneath you. Pull your arms back as if you are pulling the medicine ball into your sternum. Pause there, and then lower the ball back to the starting position.

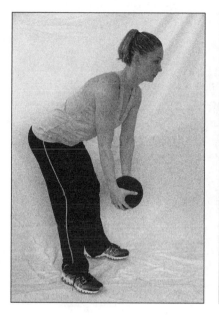
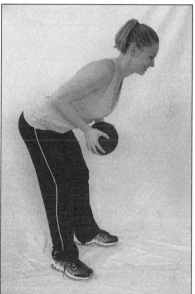

Cable Column Rows

Place an exercise cable around a column or post and step back until it straightens out. Face the column, grasp an end of the cable in each hand and lean forward, keeping your back straight. Pull the cables back as far as you can with straight arms (like a pendulum swinging) and slowly return to the starting position. For increased resistance, step farther away from the column.

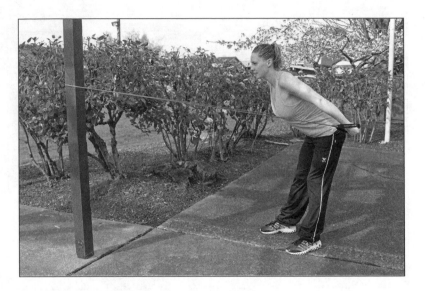

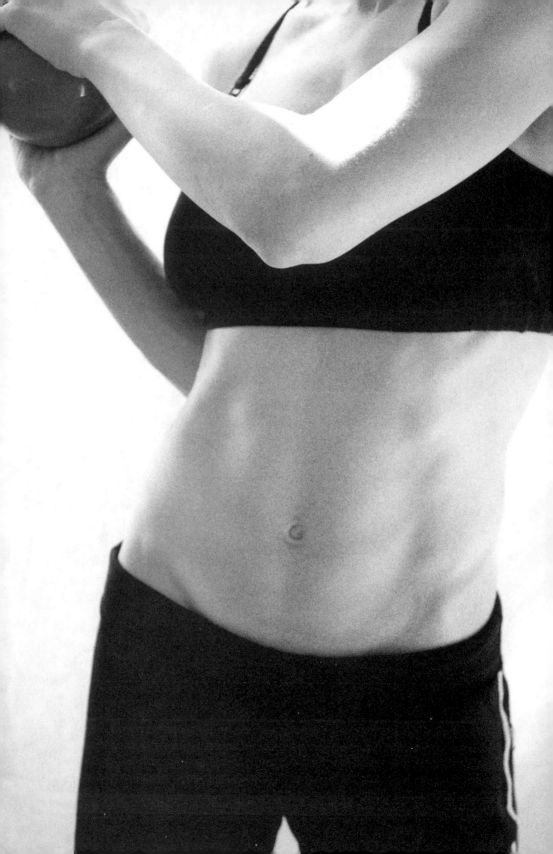

5

Core Training

When people think of core muscles they usually think of the basic abdominals: the rectus abdominis. These are the muscles that run down your center and give that six-pack look when they have been well trained and coupled with a low percentage of body fat. But there's more to the core than meets the eye. There are a variety of other important muscles just to the side of that six-pack. Specifically, you have the external and internal oblique muscles, the transverse abdominis, and spinal erectors. All of these muscles are important to build a complete physique, but there are other reasons to ensure you give the core muscles plenty of training attention.

Why Train My Core?

The biggest benefit to training the muscles of your body core is safety, not aesthetics. While it's great to have an appealing stomach for the summer and beyond, a striking physique isn't the main reason we train our abs and other muscles.

Think about the simple, everyday movements you make: getting out of a chair or sitting down in one, reaching up for something on a high shelf or reaching down to a low one, getting in or out of your car, putting on make-up, brushing your teeth, or picking up your child. What do they all have in common? They all require the use of core muscles. Strong core muscles can prevent a litany of problems in your life now and in the future.

Studies have shown that 80 to 90 percent of adults will experience significant low back pain in their lifetimes. The Bureau of Labor Statistics found that in 2010, sprains, strains, and tears made up 40 percent of the total injury claims that required days off from work. Of those, almost 40 percent were injuries related to the back.

Having a strong core can help you withstand certain types of trauma and other injuries, and strong and flexible muscles can put you at a much lower risk of those sprains, strains, and tears in any muscle group in your body. Strong core muscles can also improve your balance. So while proper training of your abs, back/lumbar, and hips can give you better aesthetics, the most important thing it provides is a safer level of functioning in everything you do!

So the question shouldn't be "Why should I train my core?" It should only be, "Why haven't I been training my core?"

Core Myths

People tend to believe a number of myths about training the abdominals and obliques. I want to clear the air right now, not only for your own good, but also for the benefit of your friends if they try to spread misinformation. You'll be able to correct them and help them get started with a better training program.

Myth #1: Crunches can hurt your neck and back. For years and years the accepted practice for abdominal training was to place your toes under something solid, lean back, put your hands behind your head, and crunch away.

Then, in time, someone wised up and realized perhaps that wasn't the safest way to do them. And while it's true that crunches with your hands behind your neck can be harmful, crunches in general aren't inherently bad for you.

Crunches, when done properly, can be great for training your abs. It's not any more appropriate to say they're dangerous than it is to say driving is dangerous. It can be, sure, but there are safe and effective ways to do it.

You should do crunches with an upward motion, not a forward motion, and you shouldn't place your hands behind your head.

Myth #2: Training my abs will make me look fat. Muscles make parts of your body bigger, right? So the theory, then, is that if you train your abdominals too much that your gut will look bigger and, thus, fatter. While strength training does increase the size of a muscle, you don't need to worry about your abs getting too big. That's because the type of exercises in this book are high-repetition, low-resistance movements that will build strength and functional safety rather than build big, bulky abs.

Working your abs won't make you look fat. Guaranteed.

Myth #3: Training obliques will make me look fat. This myth stems from the bodybuilding crowd. The theory here is that if you train your obliques—the muscles on the sides of your core—that they will start to distend outward. If you weren't worried enough about your gut hiding your shoes from all those crunches (see Myth #2), now you're wondering whether your jeans will still fit if you develop muscular obliques? It's nonsense. Doing twists and leans that strengthen your obliques will not make you look fat. But they will make your muscles more adaptable and prepared next time you have to turn around to get something.

Core Training

Even people who work out regularly often overlook proper technique when it comes to training their core. But don't worry—it's not complicated. If you read through the exercises carefully and take a long look at the pictures, you'll have these workouts down in no time.

Abdominals and Obliques

It takes a steady diet of healthy eating to get your body fat low enough for your abs to show. When combined with the right diet, these exercises will get your body built from the front so that when your shirt comes off, you'll be proud of the work you're showing off.

Standard Crunches

Sit with your toes underneath something solid—like a couch or chair—and bend at the knees so your butt is comfortable near your heels. Lean back so your back is flat on the floor, and either cross your arms over your body and each other or bring your hands up to the sides of your face.

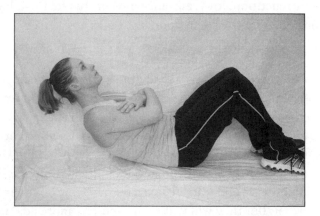

Keep your head and neck in line with your spine and draw your body toward the ceiling, *not* your knees. Pause when you reach the highest point you can comfortably go, and slowly lower yourself just above the starting position.

Ball Crunches

Sit on the exercise ball and position your feet wider than your shoulders and flat on the floor. Lean back so that you're horizontal to the ground and curl *upward,* ensuring that your feet never move.

To make this exercise even more challenging, bring your feet closer together.

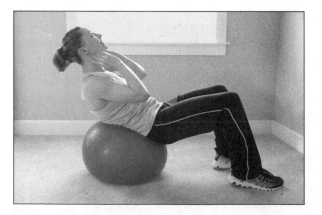

Rotating Crunches

From the standard crunch position, raise your back off the ground a few inches so that your abs are tight. Instead of continuing upward/downward and doing the normal sit-up, take both hands and reach out to the left as far as you can and touch the ground with your fingertips. Then swing your arms up and over you to your right side and touch the ground with your fingertips there as well. Touching both sides equals one rep.

You can make this increasingly difficult by creating three touch points on each side. First, touch barely outside the body on both sides, then a mid point on both sides, and then touch with your arms fully extended.

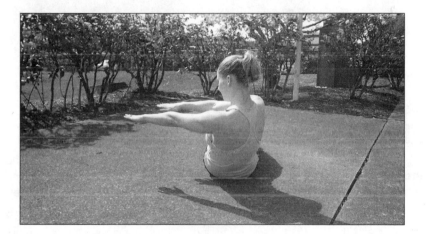

Vertical Crunches

Start flat on your back and raise your legs so they are perpendicular to your body and close together. Fold your arms over your chest and crunch your body up toward your toes while keeping your legs as still as possible.

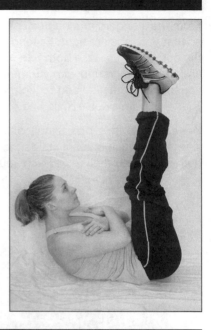

Leg Lifts

Lie flat on your back with your legs together and extended. Place your hands underneath your butt, and lift your heels about three inches from the ground. From this position raise your heels up until you feel your abdominals entirely contract and then lower them slowly to the starting position.

You can make this more challenging by extending your arms overhead (think about making your body *longer*) while lifting your legs.

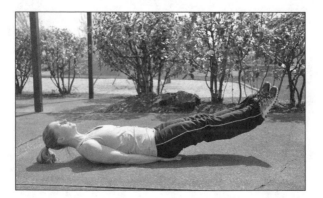

Scissor Kicks

Lie flat on your back with your legs together and extended, your hands under your butt, and your heels raised about six inches off the ground (a few inches higher than for Leg Lifts). Now, point your toes, and slowly alternate bringing one foot up while the other goes down in a scissoring motion.

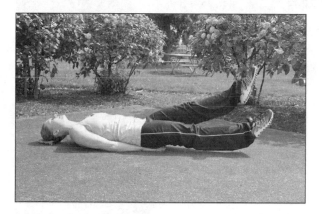

Knee Bends

From the Leg Lift position—flat on your back, legs together and extended, hands under your butt—bring your heels three to five inches off the ground. Pull your knees back toward your face as far as you can, pause there, and then extend your legs back out to the starting position.

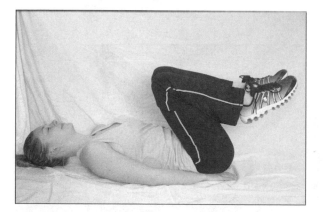

Single-Knee Bends

This is a twist on the Knee Bends. The simple difference is that instead of doing them with both legs at once, alternate legs, one knee at a time.

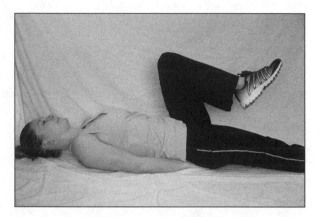

Couch Lifts

This is a great beginner's exercise for those new to training. You can use a couch, chair, bench, or even a coffee table if it suits you.

Lie with your back on the floor, your thighs vertical, and your legs bent so that, from the knee down, your legs are flat on the piece of furniture. Now, simply extend your legs straight upward before gently returning them to the starting position.

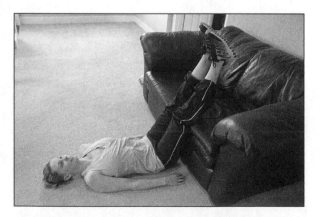

Couch Rolls

Rolls are an extension of the Couch Lift. Start in the same position, with your thighs vertical and your knees bent so that your calves rest on the piece of furniture. Extend the legs up and straight and roll backwards slightly so that your toes end up above you in line with your head, tightening your abs entirely before returning to the starting position.

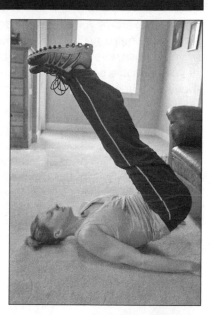

V-Ups

Lying on your back with your body fully extended from head to toe—legs straight, arms lengthened above your head—bend at the core so that your toes and fingertips come together above you. Pause at the top and slowly lower yourself back to the starting position.

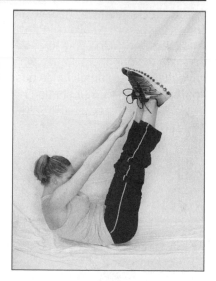

Hanging Leg Raises

This is an exercise you can easily do on playground monkey bars or, depending on your house, even from a door frame. All you need is a solid object you can grip above your head.

Hold yourself off of the ground with your arms straight above you, maintaining a slight bend in your elbows. Your hands can be gripping forward or backward, depending on what's comfortable for you. Keeping your torso still and your legs slightly bent, extend your feet straight out in front of you, pause, then slowly lower them back to the starting position.

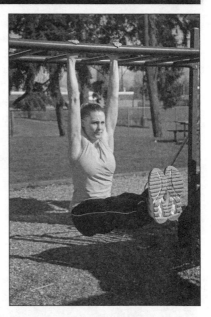

Hanging Knee Bends

Just as in Hanging Leg Raises, allow yourself to hang from a solid object with your legs extended. Bend your knees and draw them up to your chest. Pause when you have pulled them up as far as possible, and then return to your starting position.

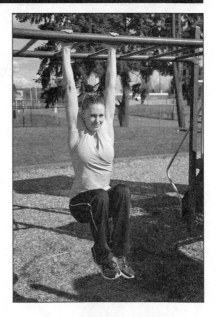

Flat Planks

Lie face down on the floor and prop yourself up on your elbows so that your body is supported only by the balls of your feet, elbows, and forearms, keeping your back straight in one solid line. Hold this position as long as possible.

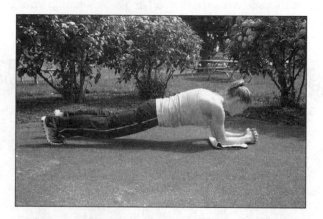

Tall Planks

Take a push-up position in which you're balanced on the balls of your feet and your hands with your arms extended. Hold this position, keeping your abs tight.

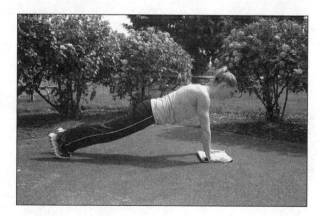

Plank Lifts

From the Flat Plank position, space your feet apart slightly. One leg at a time, lift a foot off the ground as if you are trying to touch the ceiling with the back of your heel. Pause at the height of your lift and then return to the starting position.

You can perform this same exercise on an angle by keeping your elbows and forearms propped on an exercise ball.

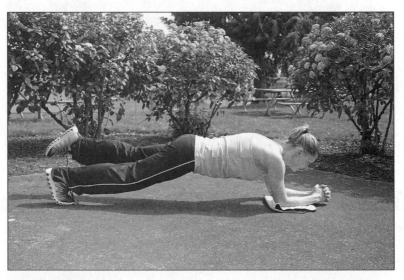

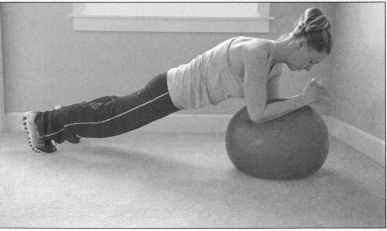

Side Planks

Position yourself on one side with your legs stacked together. Prop yourself up so that you're supported by your elbow and the side of one foot and your body is straight (no droop anywhere along the body). Hold this position, keeping your abs tight.

You can change the tension slightly by placing your elbow on an exercise ball and holding your side plank there.

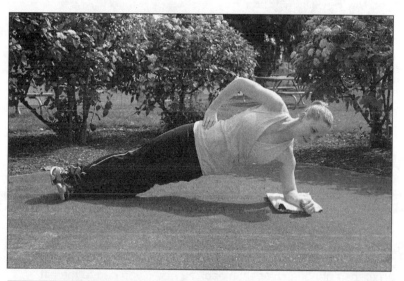

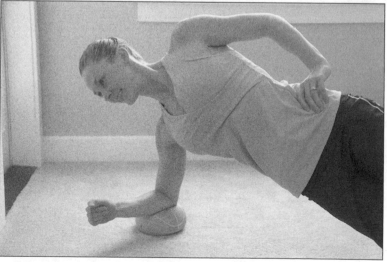

Elevated Side Planks

This is a variation of the side plank. The difference is that you elevate your legs on a couch or chair.

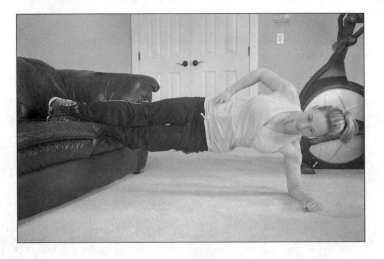

Walking Planks

With your feet elevated on a fitness ball, chair, or couch and your hands in a push-up position out on the floor in front of you, move one hand to the other, then move that hand further out. Repeat this movement until you walk as far as you can to the right of a chair, then back as far as you can to the left.

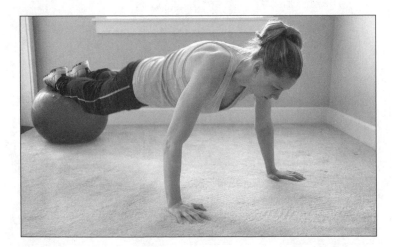

Push-Up Walk-Outs

Start in a push-up position with your hands aligned with your shoulders (close to a triceps push-up stance). One hand at a time and alternating hands, slowly move your hands forward as if you were walking forward. When your body is very close to the ground, walk hands back to the starting position.

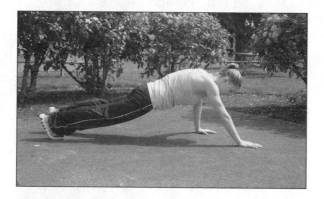

Rotating Planks

Start in a standard push-up position. Shift your weight so that you're supporting yourself with one arm, and raise the other arm straight up so that it points toward the ceiling. Keep your core tight, pause, and then return to the starting position. You can do repetitions with one arm before rotating, or you may alternate sides one by one.

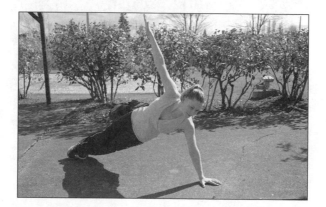

Cable Oblique Bends

Stand on a cable with one leg and hold the handle on the same side of your body so that there is a comfortable amount of tension. Keeping your spine rigid, lean to the side opposite of the hand that's holding the cable. Pause at the depth of your lean, and then return to standing tall.

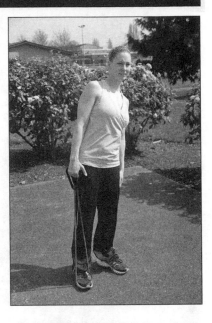

Medicine Ball Sit-Ups

Lie on your back with your knees bent up above your hips, holding a medicine ball off the ground between your feet. Place your hands at the side of your head, and crunch to bring your elbows to your knees.

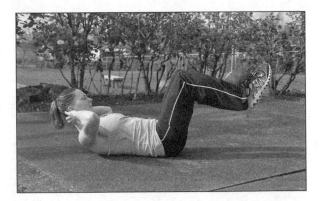

Medicine Ball Chin Sit-Ups

Lie on the ground and place your toes under the edge of a couch. Hold a medicine ball just under your chin and bring your upper body toward the ceiling. Pause at the peak, and then slowly lower yourself back to the starting position.

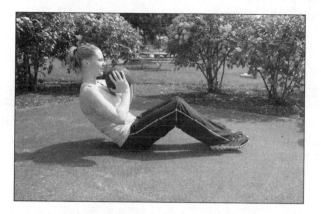

Medicine Ball Turns

With a medicine ball in your hands, stand and extend the ball at arms' length in front of you. Slowly twist your body and turn the ball to your left, then to the right, and continue back and forth.

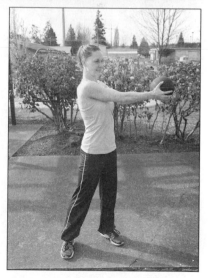

Lower Back/Hips/Glutes

It's not possible to overstate the importance of working your lower back and hips, not just from an aesthetic standpoint but even more so for safety purposes. When you move, your hips move with you. When you sit, stand, or carry things, you're counting on your lower back to be strong and limber. These exercises here not only enhance your health but your safety and comfort.

Arm Lifts

Lie on the floor face down with your arms extended in front of you. Keeping your torso, legs, and feet in contact with the ground, lift your upper body as high as you can. At your peak, pause, and then slowly lower yourself down.

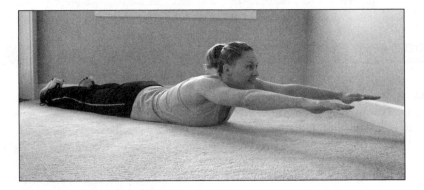

Leg Lifts

Lie face down and flat on the ground with your arms extended in front of you and your elbows and legs both bent slightly. Lift your legs as high as you can, as if you're trying to touch your heels to the ceiling. Pause at your peak, and then return to the starting position.

As an alternative, you can do a One-Leg Lift by raising just one leg at a time. You can alternate every repetition or you can do a full set with one leg and then switch to the other for an equal number of repetitions.

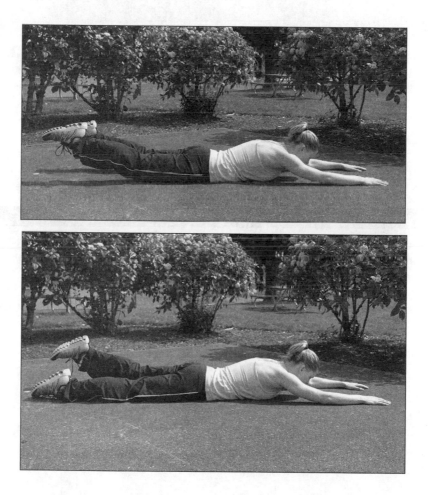

Leg Sways

This is a different take on the leg lifts just covered. With leg sways, you place your hands at a comfortable position near your sides—such as to the sides of your chest—and then raise your legs a couple of inches off the ground. Next, slowly move your legs as far as you can to your left, pause, and then move them as far as you can to your right. Sway gently left and right in equal numbers for a set or for a specific period of time.

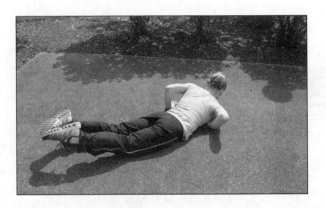

Leg Presses

Lie on your back and bend at your knees so that your feet are flat on the ground. Press down with your heels so that you lift your midsection off of the ground. Pause at the peak, and then return gently to the starting position.

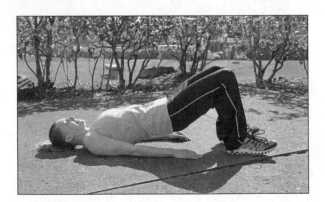

Bridges

Lie on your back and bend at the knees until your feet are flat on the ground. Bring your arms straight up above you and bend them at the elbows so that your hands are next to your head, palms down, with fingers pointing toward your toes. Press yourself up into the shape of a bridge, pause at the peak, and return to the starting position.

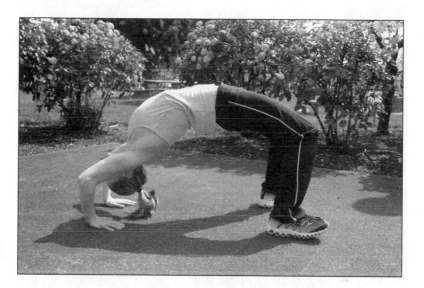

Hip Twists

Lie on your back and extend your arms out to your sides with your palms flat. Bend your knees so that they come up toward your chest, keeping your legs together. Rotate your hips to your left, pause, then back over to the right, pausing again, before bringing them back to the starting position.

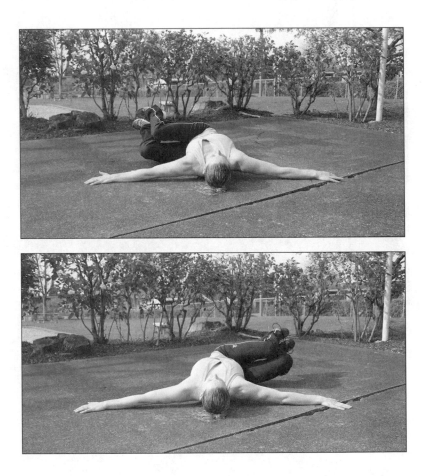

Side Leg Lifts

Lie on your side with your legs stacked one on top of the other. You can prop yourself up on an arm or lie flat. Lift one leg toward the ceiling as high as possible, pause, then lower it until it's an inch or two above the starting position, and then raise it again. Repeat the movement with the opposite leg.

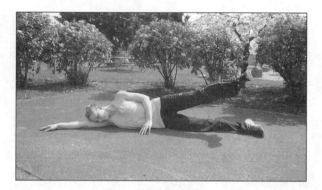

Hip Draws

From a push-up position, draw one knee up underneath and across your body as far as you can, aiming for the opposite elbow. Place leg back in the starting position and repeat the movement with the opposite leg.

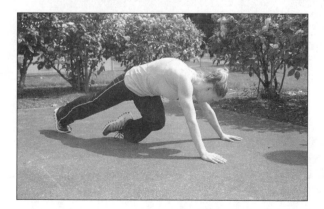

Hip Turns

Starting in a traditional push-up position, bring one knee up to your chest as far as you can, lift it up to your side as high as possible, and then return to the starting position. You can repeat for reps with one leg before alternating legs, or alternate back and forth.

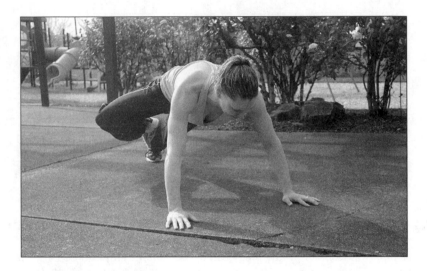

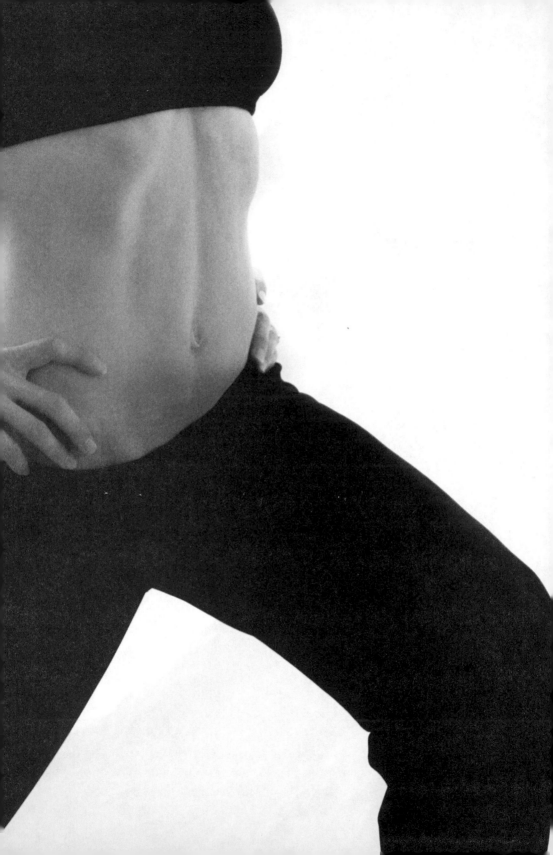

6

Lower Body Training

Whether you're walking around the mall, mowing the lawn, doing laundry, or getting out of a chair, having well-trained legs makes life much easier. You may have noticed in the past that walking around a county fair or even the grocery store makes your legs tired; after doing these exercises for even a short period of time, you won't worry about that any longer.

Many people don't think about legs when they train. Plenty of people who train only work on their chests and arms because those are the aesthetic muscles. But your legs are the foundation of your body. Even if you work with your hands, you still need strong and balanced legs to achieve maximum efficiency. Give your legs ample attention when you work out, and you'll find your body as a whole feels better as well as looks better. Firming up those legs—getting rid of any "jiggle" you may have—will boost your confidence and keep you motivated.

And, as if you needed more reasons to realize the importance of leg training, science has shown that, because of the size of the muscles in the legs and the amount of blood within them, intense leg training can increase the amount of growth hormone that, ultimately, helps your *entire body* burn fat more efficiently and add muscle!

Quadriceps

The upper leg is broken up into two main muscles: the quadriceps and the hamstrings. The quadriceps are the large muscles you see on the front of your legs; give them ample attention to maximize your leg strength.

Squats

Place your legs just beyond shoulder-width with your toes pointed relatively straight. Rest your hands at your hips, keep your spine straight, and slowly lower yourself until your thighs are horizontal to the ground. Pause there, then push yourself back to the starting position.

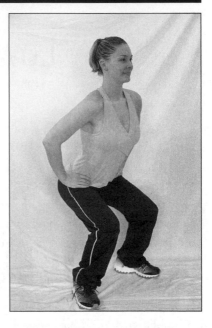

You can also do this exercise while holding a medicine ball or exercise ball. Raise the ball above your head as you squat down and bring it down and hold it out in front of you as you stand.

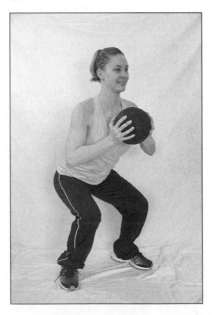

Squat Holds

Take a squat position and lower yourself until your thighs are horizontal to the
ground. Hold this position for as long as
you can.

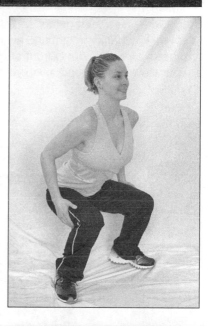

Exercise Ball Wall Squats

Place an exercise ball behind your back
and lean against a wall, so that the ball is
between you and the wall. Stand with feet
just beyond shoulder-width apart, slowly
lower yourself down until your thighs are
parallel to the ground, and then push yourself back up.

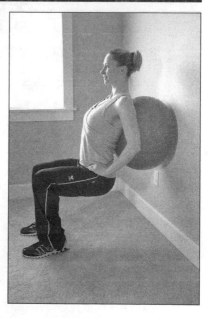

Close-Knee Squats

Stand with your feet together and slowly lower yourself down into a squat, keeping your back straight and avoiding leaning forward. You may find it useful to place your hands out in front of you to assist in balancing. When your thighs are parallel to the ground, push yourself back to the starting position.

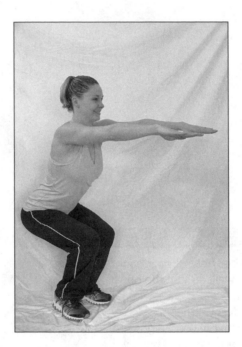

Knee Drops

Form your body into a V-shape by placing your hands on the ground and your feet just a couple of feet behind you with your butt in the air. Keeping your head in line with the body, bend your knees until they are just barely off the ground and you're balancing on your hands and the balls of your feet, and then return to the starting position.

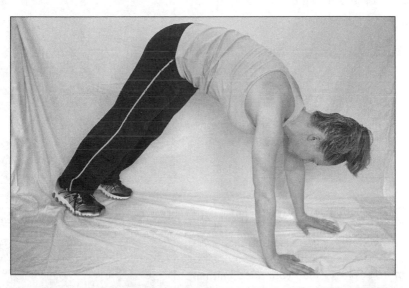

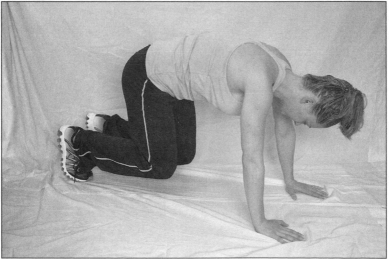

Lunges

Stand with your feet side by side and your knees slightly bent. With one leg, take a medium step forward and bend at the knee until your back knee nearly touches the floor. From this position, either step forward with the back leg and repeat the process, or return to the starting position and alternate legs.

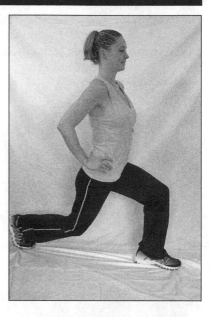

One-Leg Chair Squats

Balance yourself on one leg and place the other leg's heel up on the seat of a chair or flat, sturdy object Place your hands either on your hips or extended out in front of you, and bend at the knee of the leg you're standing on. Squat as deeply as you can, pause, then push yourself back to the starting position.

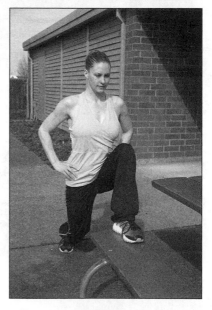

Step-Ups

Using a sturdy chair or bench, step up onto it and slowly lower yourself back down.

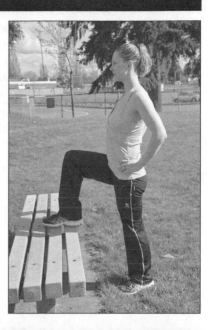

Squat Jumps

Stand with your feet just beyond shoulder-width and your knees slightly bent. Keeping your hands in front of you but near your chest, squat down as far as you can and then explosively push off of your feet and jump into the air. Bring your knees as high as you can in the air before landing, going right into your next squat.

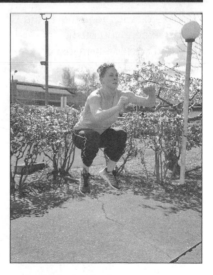

Chair Squats

Sit in a chair with your back straight and feet flat on the floor. Extend both arms out in front of you and then push from your heels and stand up without leaning forward.

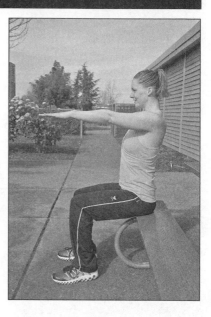

One-Leg Chair Squats

This exercise is the same as the Chair Squat, except you push yourself into standing position with just one leg. The body's natural tendency is to lean forward, but try not to.

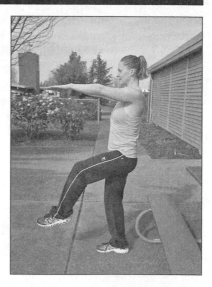

Leaning Squats

Stand with your feet outside of shoulder-width and your hands up in front of your chest or at your sides. Bend the knee of one leg until your quadricep is parallel to the ground, or as far as is comfortable, then push yourself over onto the other side and repeat.

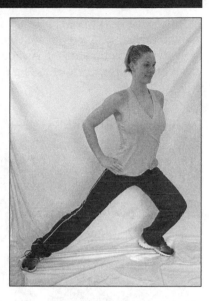

Rotating Lunges

Stand and hold a medicine ball in front of your chest. Step forward with one leg and lower yourself into a standard lunge, keeping the medicine ball at your chest. When you're in the lowered position, turn your torso—keeping the medicine ball in the same place—from left to right and then back facing forward. Return to the starting position or step into the next lunge with the other leg.

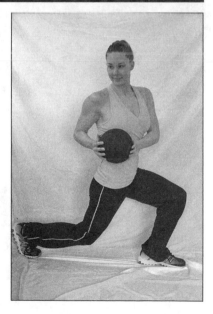

Medicine Ball Squat-Presses

This exercise is for your shoulders as well as your legs. Take a medicine ball in hand and keep it near your chest. Bend at the knees and squat down, and then stand back up straight. As you stand, extend the ball above you, and then lower it back down to the starting position.

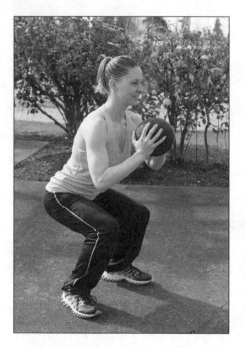 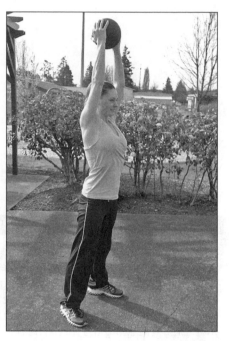

Hamstrings

Although they don't tend to get as much attention because you can't see them, the hamstrings are a vitally important muscle group to train. They make up the back portion of your thighs and are involved whenever you bend at the knees or even when you bend forward.

One-Leg Chair Dips

Place a sturdy chair about two feet behind you, bend the knee of one leg back behind you, and rest the top of that foot on the seat. Slowly bend the leg you're standing on, going as deeply as you can. Pause there, then push yourself back to the starting position.

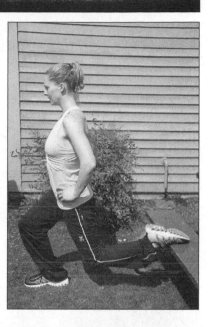

Half Bridges

Lie face-up on the floor with your knees bent so your feet are flat on the floor. Pressing your feet into the ground, bring your butt and hips toward the ceiling until your heels come off the ground and you are on the tips of your toes. Pause and slowly lower to the ground.

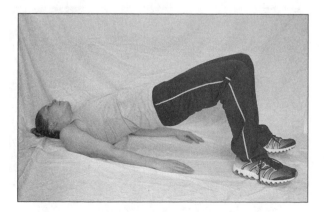

One-Leg Half Bridges

This is the same as the Half Bridge, but before pressing yourself up, extend one leg straight. Use only one leg to press yourself up and onto the ball of that foot, then slowly lower back down.

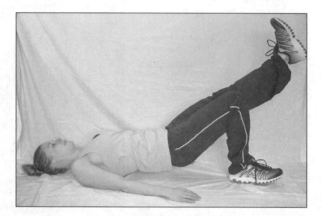

One-Leg Elevated Bridges

Lie face-up with your back on the floor and your heels resting on an elevated platform such as a chair, couch, or sturdy coffee table. Lift one leg while keeping the other heel in place, and then lift your hips off of the ground as high as you can.

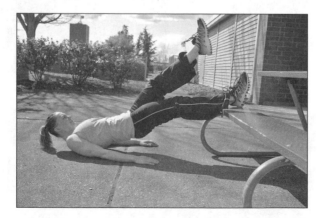

Elevated Bridges

This is the same exercise as the One-Leg Elevated Bridge, but you keep both of your heels on the elevated surface as you raise your hips.

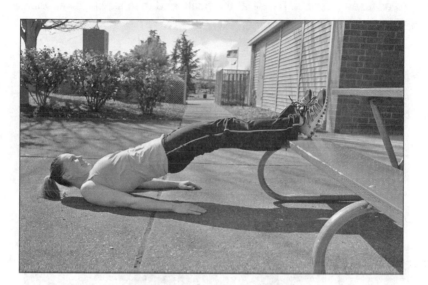

Hamstring Lifts

Sit on the floor with your hands flat on the floor, fingertips pointing ahead of you. Position your hands slightly behind your back, and point your toes. In a smooth motion, push into your heels and use your hamstrings to lift your hips upward as far as possible. Pause at the peak, and then slowly lower yourself back down.

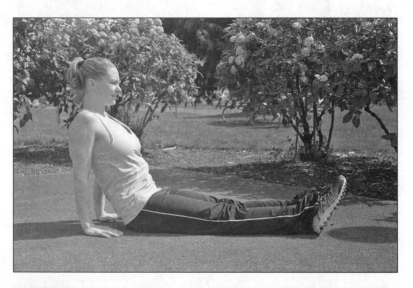

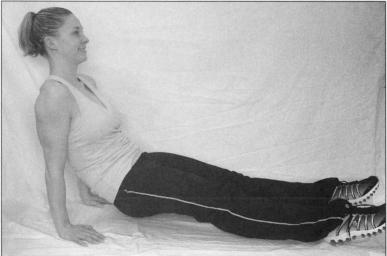

Exercise Ball Hamstring Curls

Lie face-up with your back on the floor. Place an exercise ball under your calves with your legs straight. Bend your knees and roll your feet onto the ball, lifting your hamstrings and butt off of the ground, and then roll the ball back out.

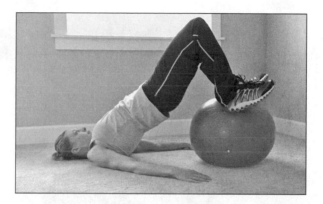

Hamstring Leans

Stand with your back straight and lean forward from the waist, letting one leg rise up behind you (keeping it straight). Reach down to the toe of the foot that's on the floor, continuing to lean forward until you are parallel to the ground from heel to head. Repeat for opposite leg.

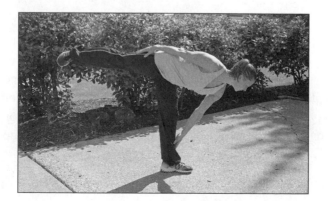

Medicine Ball Lifts

Stand with your knees slightly bent and hold a medicine ball in front of your legs with your arms straight. Slowly lean forward, keeping your back straight, and slide the medicine ball down in front of you until it reaches the top of your feet, and then slowly stand back up.

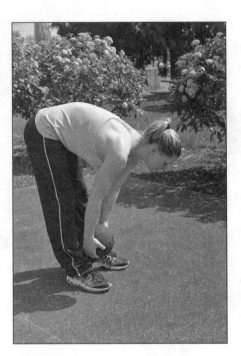

Calves

The calves are a notoriously stubborn body part to train, but because they come into play in varying degrees anytime you have ankle flexion—such as with every step you take—they're worth giving some attention to when you're training. Although a small muscle group, they play an important role both functionally and aesthetically in the leg make-up.

Calf Raises on a Stair

Place the balls of your feet on the end of a stair so your heels hang over the edge. Lower yourself down as far as possible, and then push up until you are standing as tall as possible on the balls of your feet. Pause at the peak, and then slowly lower yourself back down.

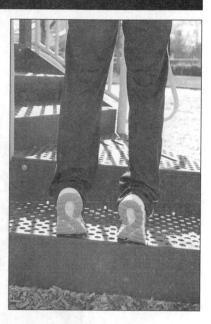

You can do variations of this exercise by turning your toes out to a "10 and 2" position (corresponding to the numbers on the face of a clock).

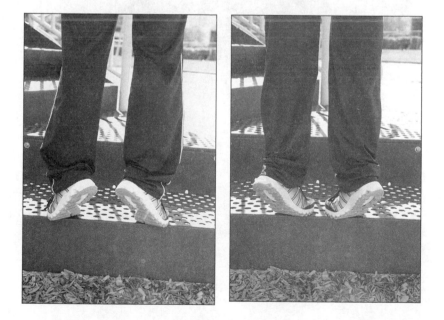

One-Leg Calf Raises

As with the regular calf raise, place the ball of your foot on the step with your heel hanging over the edge. Place the opposite leg around the back of the leg you will be exercising, then lower yourself as far as possible, and then push up as high as possible. Switch legs and repeat.

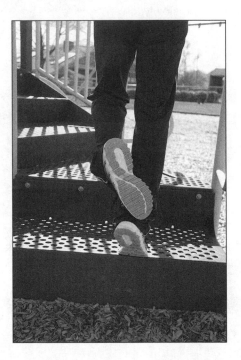

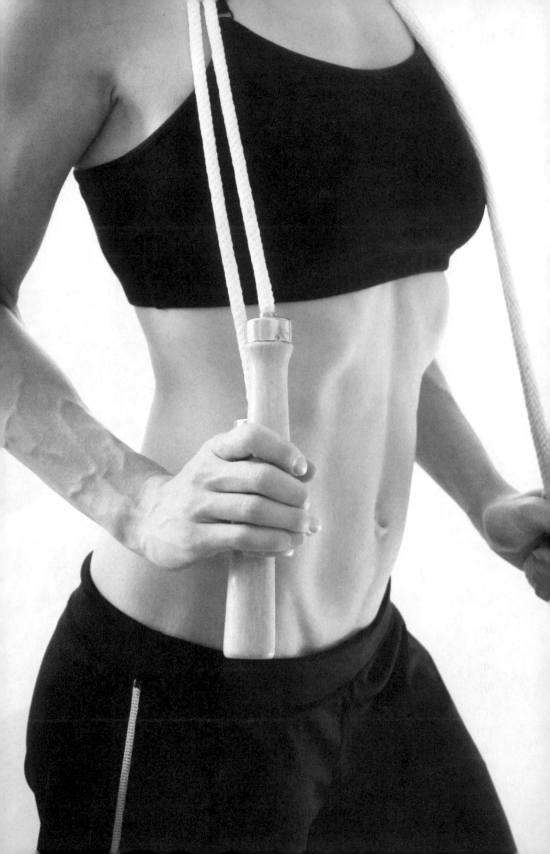

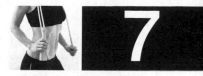

7

Breathing Easier:
Cardiovascular Exercise

Cardiovascular exercise, or simply cardio for short, is any activity that increases your heart rate from its base rate. Cardiovascular exercise improves your overall health. From helping to burn extra calories to lowering your blood pressure, you have a litany of reasons to get moving and get your heart rate up.

The Benefits of Cardio

Often, when people think of cardio, they think of running. And although running is an ideal cardiovascular activity, there are a lot of other activities that can get your heart going and create a little sweat. With every step, stair, climb, or reach—techniques you can use in various cardiovascular activities—you'll be moving in the direction of better health and happiness.

Science-Backed Studies

Being active and increasing your heart rate for sustained periods of time is important. But people don't seem to understand just *how* important. So, to put it into perspective and make clear how even just going for a walk can improve the quality and length of your life, here's a look at a few studies:

In 2002, the *New England Journal of Medicine* published a study that looked at the effects of exercise, ranging from walking to more vigorous cardio, on women. They concluded that walking and more intense cardio exercise are *both* associated with substantial reductions in heart-related health problems, regardless of race, age, or weight. Further, they found that extended periods of a sedentary lifestyle increased cardiovascular risk.

Aside from physical health benefits, cardiovascular activities provide mental benefits, too. In 2005, the publication *Current Opinion in Psychiatry* found that exercise and sustained physical activity improved mental health. These improvements were found in diverse ethnic populations, in both men and women, and for people of all ages.

To tack on to the brain benefits, in 2009, *Neuropsychological Rehabilitation: An International Journal* published results of a study that shows aerobic endurance exercise was largely beneficial to memory in young adults, both boys and girls. Additionally, in 2006 the *Annals of Internal Medicine* published the results of a study that showed a year-long exercise program was highly beneficial to the memories of adults of all ages, and greatly reduced the risk of dementia in adults over 65.

So, as you can see, from your mind all the way down to the muscles in your feet, cardiovascular exercise will improve your life. The key is finding something you enjoy—because you'll only stick with a cardio program if you enjoy it!

What's Considered Cardio

Running is certainly considered cardio, but so is swimming, stair climbing, or even taking a walk. You can get the benefits of cardiovascular exercise by doing anything that increases your heart rate from its base rate. Here are some sports and other activities that have a considerable cardio component:

> Basketball
>
> Bicycling
>
> Jogging
>
> Skating
>
> Soccer
>
> Squash
>
> Swimming
>
> Tennis
>
> Water Polo

Your cardio doesn't have to come from a sport, though. And you certainly don't need to go to a gym to get a good cardio workout. Even daily activities like walking your dog can be considered cardiovascular as long as you do it vigorously enough to raise your heart rate. Other ways to increase your cardio include walking stairs at work instead of taking the elevator, mowing your lawn with a push mower, and even romping with your kids.

Target Heart Rate

How do you know whether you're working hard enough for your activity to constitute a cardiovascular workout? It's actually fairly simple: you want to maintain a rate of about 70 percent of your maximum heart rate. To determine your maximum heart rate (MHR), subtract your age from 220. If you're 25, your presumed MHR is 195 (220 – 25 = 195). And while interval training (in which you find yourself getting close to your MHR number for brief periods before returning to an easier pace) is beneficial from time to time, for general fitness it is recommended that you maintain a rate of about 70 percent of your MHR during the majority of your cardio.

If you've never taken your heart rate, you can easily do so by feeling your pulse (in your wrist using the two fingers of the opposite hand, or in your neck just to the side of the throat) and count for 10 seconds. Multiply that number by six, and there you have it.

Passing the Time

One of the most common excuses I hear for why people don't do cardio training is that it's boring. One way to avoid boredom is to choose an activity that you're passionate about. If you like what you're doing, you'll be engaged in it, and the time will seem to fly by.

You can also avoid boredom by listening to music or a good book while you're working out. Long gone are the days you had to bring along a bulky Walkman. Now, with an mp3 player—a device smaller than a credit card— you can listen to music, audio books, or a language-learning program. Of course, if you have a smartphone, you can even listen to an internet stream from a program like Pandora or your favorite podcast.

By all means, if it's feasible, feel free to invest in something that will take your mind off exercise. Mp3 players are great technology and you can't help but think they were made for the fitness enthusiast.

Another way to pass the time while you're exercising is to do it with a friend. Since you should only be shooting for about 70 percent of your maximum heart rate, you should be able to carry on a conversation while you train. By focusing on the conversation rather than the workout, the time will seem to fly by.

Getting Moving

Not everyone likes old-fashioned methods of cardiovascular exercise. If you count yourself in this category, don't beat yourself up. Running isn't for everyone, whether that's because you just don't enjoy it or perhaps it's too painful for your knees or other joints. Additionally, bad weather can often adversely affect one's desire to work out outside. And when it comes to sports like tennis or basketball, you may have trouble finding someone with the same schedule to play against. So if you're by yourself or just want variety, I describe a variety of cardio exercises in the pages that follow.

If you enjoy steady-state cardio (such as running, biking, etc.) by all means continue to enjoy those, but I encourage you to give these movements a try just for variety.

The following are a list of cardiovascular exercises that I include in the circuits in Chapter 8. While each could be used continually on its own, putting them together in varied amounts of time gives you a much more complete training experience. Practice each technique before trying it in a circuit or workout to make sure you've got the technique down and that it's comfortable for you.

Star Picker

Stand tall with your arms bent at the elbow so your hands are up about face height and your palms are facing out. Staying light on the balls of your feet, bring one knee up high and, as you do, reach up with the opposite arm (when you raise your left knee, extend your right arm, and vice versa). Continually alternate sides.

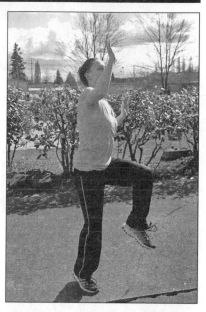

Star Jumps

Squat down as far as you can with your feet together and your arms close to your body. From this position, explode upward in a jumping motion and throw your arms and legs out to the sides to form an X-like shape. As you land softly, draw your arms and legs back in, squat back down, and repeat.

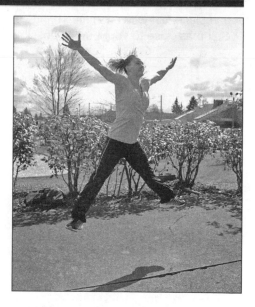

High Knees

This exercise is similar to running in place: alternate bringing your knees as close to your chest as possible, pumping your arms up and down at your sides as you go.

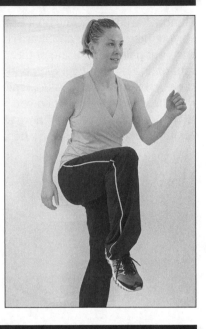

Butt Kicking

Jog in place, but with each step bring your heels up as close to your butt as possible.

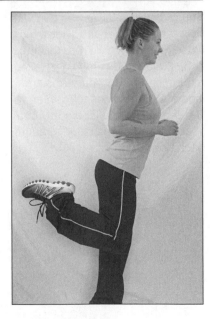

Ski Jumps

Stand with your legs together, bend your knees, and lean your chest forward slightly. Keep your arms at your sides and draw your hands up toward your chest. Using your legs, jump to one side, landing softly on the balls of your feet, and then jump back to the other side.

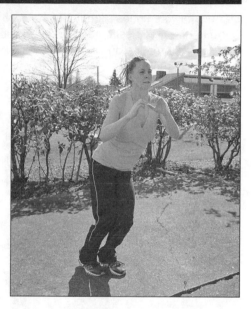

Toe Kicks

Stand with your knees slightly bent and your arms held out to your sides. Begin by making circling motions with your arms and hop up by pushing off on the balls of your feet, alternating one leg at a time. With the non-hopping leg kick forward slightly, as if you're flicking off a shoe. As you hop, alternate foot.

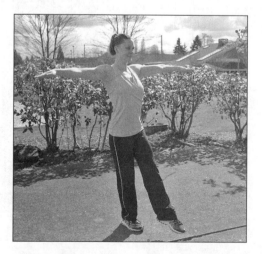

Crossovers

Stand with your knees slightly bent and your arms crossed over the body as if you're giving yourself a really big hug. Hop up by pushing off on the balls of your feet, alternating one leg at a time. As you hop, open your arms wide and throw them back across, alternating which arm is on top with each repetition.

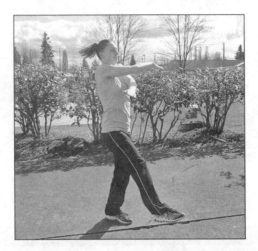

Dual Squats

Stand with your feet just beyond shoulder-width apart. Squat down until your thighs are parallel to the ground, and then powerfully push yourself upward and jump into the air, bringing your legs together as soon as your feet clear the ground. Land on the balls of your feet, and then squat down again. When you push back off, jump high into the air once again, land back in the wide stance, and repeat.

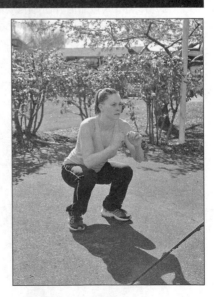

Side Steps

You've probably seen this exercise in magazine articles featuring easy workouts. It's a great warm up for your lower body and hips. Start by taking a wide step to your left and then bringing the right foot to the left, then stepping out wide with the right foot and repeating the process with the left. You'll end up bouncing back and forth, side to side. You can keep your arms at your sides or swing them forward with each step.

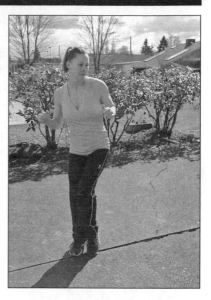

Long Leaps

Stand with your feet together and your knees slightly bent. Push off of the ground and place one leg as far out in front as possible while the opposite leg goes behind you as far as is comfortable, then jump and alternate legs. Pump your arms back and forth as you continue alternating legs.

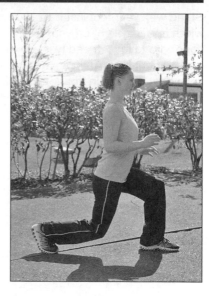

Jumping Jacks

Stand up straight with your feet close to-gether and your hands at your sides. Jump up and kick your legs out to your side so that when you land, your feet are just past shoulder-width apart. As you jump, swing your arms straight out and over your head until your fingertips nearly touch. Jump back to the starting position, bring your arms back down to your side as you do.

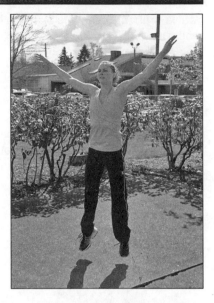

Body Twists

Stand with your feet just beyond shoulder-width and stay light on your feet. Rotate your core to the left and twist on the ball of your right foot. At the same time, swing your right arm out in front of you with an open palm toward the direction you're turning (almost like you were going to slap someone). Rotate back to your start position and repeat with the other side, continuing to alternate.

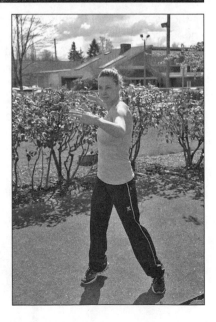

Mountain Climbers

Start in a traditional push-up position, keeping your core tight. Bring one knee up as close to your chest as possible while balancing on the opposite foot, and then quickly switch legs. Using rapid motions, continue to alternate legs.

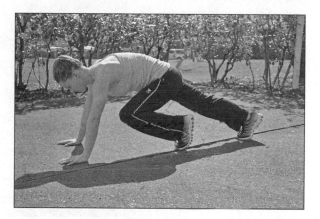

Push-Up U-Jump

Start in a traditional push-up position. Push off on your toes and bring them as close to your hands as possible, landing as softly as you can. Hop back out into the push-up position and repeat.

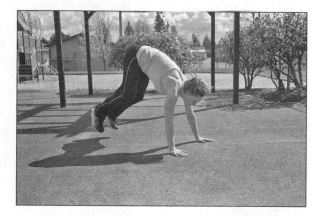

Medicine Ball Sprints

Squat down and hold a medicine ball in your hands with your arms extended down between your feet. In a smooth motion, stand to your feet and use your core strength to throw the ball as far in front of you as possible. Sprint as fast as you can to the ball, not slowing down until you reach it. Pick up the ball, run back to your original position, and repeat.

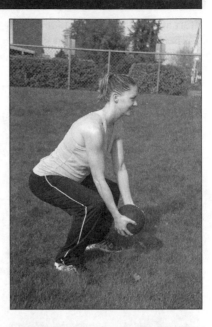

Medicine Ball Overhead Throws

Squat down while holding a medicine ball in your hands with your arms extended down between your feet. Quickly in one motion, push off the ground with your feet as you stand and jump into the air, throwing the ball as high in the air as possible. Let the ball land on the ground (make sure you avoid getting hit!), and then approach the ball, squat down, and repeat.

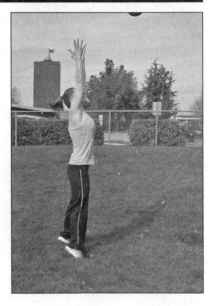

Medicine Ball Rear Throws

Squat down while holding a medicine ball in your hands with your arms extended down between your feet. With a controlled, powerful, explosive movement, quickly drive your body upward to a standing position as you throw the ball behind you as far as possible. After it lands, go to it, and repeat for reps.

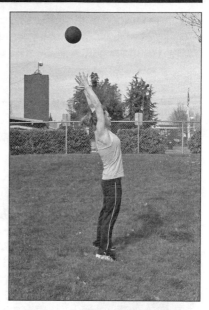

Knee Jumps

Stand up with your knees just slightly bent and your hands in a comfortable position for jumping. Staying light on your feet, jump into the air and draw your knees as close to your chest as possible.

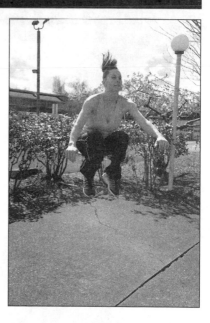

Hop Jumps

Starting in a squatting position, push off your feet as hard as possible and jump forward. Land softly on your feet and squat right back down so you can repeat the movement.

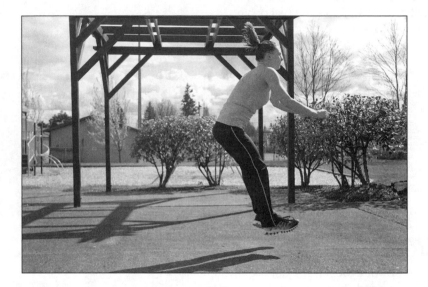

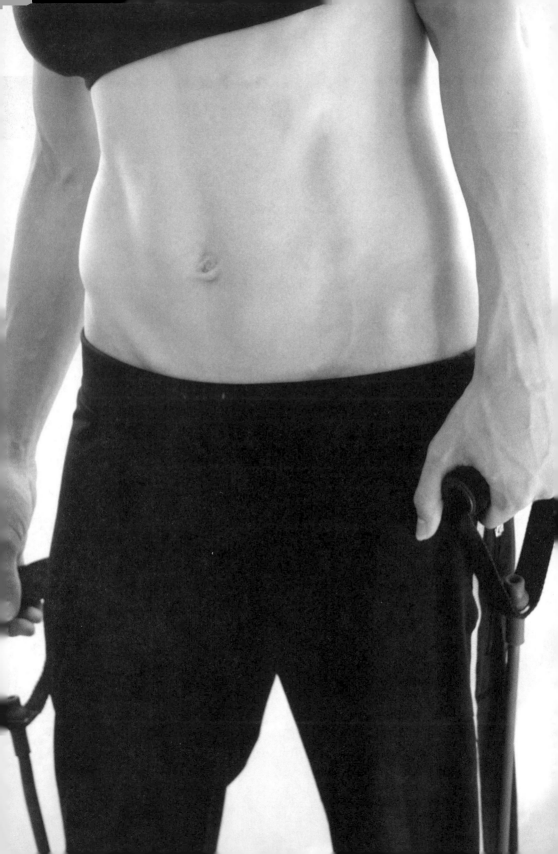

8

Ready-to-Go Workouts

You'll find in short order that your fitness program takes on a life of its own. You'll find yourself crafting new and challenging sets and, perhaps, even creating a couple of new exercises as you grow fitter, leaner, and stronger. But along the way you may prefer having some preset, ready-to-go workouts at your disposal. This chapter has everything you need for that.

In these pages you'll find workouts that tax and tone every muscle group in the body and help you achieve your goals quickly and efficiently.

How Much? How Often?

The debate will likely forever rage about how often you should work a particular muscle group. There are critics of the popular methodology to work each muscle once per week. This is often called a Bodybuilder Split. Those against it say that normal people should train their body more often than bodybuilders because they want more "functional" strength and not just muscular size. Then, of course, there is a large chorus that will gladly explain that training more than once per week is too much, and multiple efforts on a muscle group lead to overtraining.

So what is right for you? Whatever *feels* right. You may find that you can train shoulders on a Wednesday and, by Monday, they're ready to go again. If that's the case, and you're really in the mood to work them once more, go for it. On the other hand, you might train legs on a Tuesday and, by the following Wednesday, they still just don't feel fresh. If you aren't ready to squat and lunge until Thursday, that's perfectly fine, too. No one can tell you that the signals your body sends you are wrong; in fact, they're perfectly right for you. And when it comes to your workouts, you're the only person who matters!

How to Use These Workouts

These workouts are meant for you to adapt and use in sequence. The early workouts are geared toward people who haven't trained before or haven't done so in a very long time. They begin with basic, single-muscle routines and then evolve into multi-muscle circuits. Later workouts are higher volume, more intense, and aimed at experienced trainers. The workouts in the middle gradually build you up to the more advanced workouts by introducing movements and accessories to fully round out your training.

Some workouts focus on a single muscle group, while others combine two muscle groups. Further still, some workouts are directed toward an entire section of the body, such as full upper-body and lower-body workouts. I provide so many options to enable you to try a variety of routines and find what combinations work best for you. After all, by the time you're done with these workouts, my goal is for you to feel confident and comfortable with training, understand your body, and be able to craft training sequences that best fit *you*.

You are going to see the workouts noted like this:

3 × 15 Medicine Ball Lift

The '3' means three sets. The '× 15' means 15 reps during each set. For multi-set exercises with variable repetitions as the sets go on, the rep range for each set is notated as follows:

Medicine Ball Lifts

> 3 Sets
>
> - Set 1: 8 Reps
>
> - Set 2: 9 Reps
>
> - Set 3: 10 Reps

As far as frequency, feel free to start off with one training day per muscle group per week, and expand as necessary. If you find you can train more often, then go for it! If the reps listed aren't right for you, feel free to add or subtract a couple to make it suit you.

Lastly, after the workouts, I've included several cardio circuits. This is a collection of suggested routines to burn calories and fat through cardiovascular exercise. Add these in after you're comfortable with the training, and do so on as many days as you feel you have the energy. Ideally, you'll do some cardio work at least three days a week, but this may increase based on your total energy level and experience.

Keep in mind that all of these workouts assume you have properly warmed up beforehand with the same kind of techniques discussed in Chapter 3. Without further ado, let's get started!

Workouts

Workout 1: Beginning Legs

3 × 10 Squats

3 × 10 Step-Ups

3 × 12 Lunges

5 × 10 Calf Raises

Workout 2: Beginning Chest

4 × 10 Push-Ups

2 × 10 Incline Push-Ups

2 × 10 Decline Push-Ups

Workout 3: Arms and Abdominals

4 × 10 Curls

4 × 12 Triceps Dips

3 × 10 Triceps Push-Ups

4 × 15 Standard Crunches

Workout 4: Shoulders

4 × 10 Shoulder Push-Ups

3 × 12 Side Laterals

3 × 12 Rear Laterals

Workout 5: Back

3 × 15 Lying Arm Raises: Front

3 × 15 Lying Arm Raises: Side

3 × 8 Table Pulls

Workout 6: Lower Body

4 × 12 Squats

3 × 15 Knee Drops

3 × 30-second Squat Holds

5 × 15 Calf Raises

3 × 15 Leg Sways

Workout 7: Chest and Triceps

4 × 12 Incline Push-Ups

3 × 12 Dip Push-Ups

3 × 12 Triceps Push-Ups

4 × 15 Triceps Dips

Workout 8: Shoulders and Back

3 × 10 Shoulder Push-Ups

4 × 15 Rear Laterals

4 × 15 Side Laterals

3 × 12 Table Pulls

3 × 15 Lying Arm Raises: Front

3 × 15 Lying Arm Raises: Side

Workout 9: Abs and Obliques

3 × 12 Rotating Crunches

3 × 30 Scissor Kicks

4 × 15 Couch Lifts

3 × 30-second Flat Planks

3 × 30-second Side Planks

Workout 10: Chest and Shoulders

3 × 12 Dip Push-Ups

4 × 15 Push-Ups

4 × 15 Decline Push-Ups

3 × 15 Front Laterals

5 × 12 Side Laterals

4 × 12 Shoulder Push-Ups

Workout 11: Legs

3 × 45-second Squat Holds

Leaning Squats

 3 Sets

 - Set 1: 10 Reps

 - Set 2: 12 Reps

 - Set 3: 15 Reps

Knee Drops

 3 Sets

 - Set 1: 12 Reps

 - Set 2: 12 Reps

 - Set 3: 15 Reps

One-Leg Chair Dips

 4 Scts

 - Set 1: 10 Reps

 - Set 2: 10 Reps

 - Set 3: 12 Reps

 - Set 4: 12 Reps

4 × 15 Lunges

Workout 12: Arms and Back

Cable Curls

    4 Sets

    - Set 1: 10 Reps

    - Set 2: 10 Reps

    - Set 3: 15 Reps

    - Set 4: 15 Reps

3 × 12 Cable Hammer Curls

Triceps Overhead Extensions

    3 Sets

    - Set 1: 10 Reps

    - Set 2: 10 Reps

    - Set 3: 15 Reps

Triceps Cable Extensions

    3 Sets

    - Set 1: 12 Reps

    - Set 2: 12 Reps

    - Set 3: 15 Reps

Table Pulls

    4 Sets

    - Set 1: 6 Reps

    - Set 2: 7 Reps

    - Set 3: 8 Reps

    - Set 4: 10 Reps

4 × 15 Cable Column Rows

Workout 13: Shoulders, Abs, and Obliques

Shoulder Push-Ups

>   4 Sets

>   - Set 1: 7 Reps

>   - Set 2: 10 Reps

>   - Set 3: 15 Reps

>   - Set 4: 15 Reps

4 × 12 Cable Overhead Presses

Side Laterals

>   3 Sets

>   - Set 1: 12 Reps

>   - Set 2: 15 Reps

>   - Set 3: 15 Reps

3 × 20 Ball Crunches

4 × 15 Leg Lifts

3 × 45-second Elevated Side Planks

3 × 15 Cable Oblique Bends

Workout 14: Lower Body

Squats

2 Sets

- Set 1: 15 Reps

- Set 2: 20 Reps

2 × 15 Close-Knee Squats

3 × 10 One-Leg Chair Squats

3 × 15 Hamstring Lifts

Hip Lifts

3 Sets

- Set 1: 12 Reps

- Set 2: 15 Reps

- Set 3: 15 Reps

Workout 15: Chest and Calves

Cable Post Flies

> 4 Sets
>
> - Set 1: 10 Reps
>
> - Set 2: 12 Reps
>
> - Set 3: 15 Reps
>
> - Set 4: 18 Reps

4 × 12 Cable Chest Presses

Dip Push-Ups

> 3 Sets
>
> - Set 1: 10 Reps
>
> - Set 2: 10 Reps
>
> - Set 3: 12 Reps

Plyometric Push-Ups

> 2 Sets
>
> - Set 1: 4 Reps
>
> - Set 2: 6 Reps

3 × 20 Calf Raises

3 × 10 One-Leg Calf Raises

Workout 16: Shoulders and Arms

Cable Overhead Presses

    4 Sets

    - Set 1: 10 Reps

    - Set 2: 12 Reps

    - Set 3: 15 Reps

    - Set 4: 20 Reps

4×15 Rear Laterals

Front Laterals

    4 Sets

    - Set 1: 10 Reps

    - Set 2: 12 Reps

    - Set 3: 15 Reps

    - Set 4: 18 Reps

4×15 Side Laterals

5×10 Cable Curls

Medicine Ball Arm Curls

    3 Sets

    - Set 1: 10 Reps

    - Set 2: 12 Reps

    - Set 3: 12 Reps

Workout 17: Legs and Abs

Hip Draws

    3 Sets

    - Set 1: 10 Reps

    - Set 2: 12 Reps

    - Set 3: 15 Reps

4 × 15 Side Leg Lifts

4 × 15 Close-Knee Squats

Squat Jumps

    3 Sets

    - Set 1: 6 Reps

    - Set 2: 8 Reps

    - Set 3: 10 Reps

3 × 45-second Tall Planks

3 × 5 Push-Up Walk-Outs

Workout 18: Back and Obliques

Cable Column Rows

>5 Sets

>- Set 1: 12 Reps

>- Set 2: 12 Reps

>- Set 3: 15 Reps

>- Set 4: 15 Reps

>- Set 5: 20 Reps

3×15 Table Pulls

3×20 Medicine Ball Rows

Side Planks

>4 Sets

>- Set 1: 30 seconds

>- Set 2: 45 seconds

>- Set 3: 45 seconds

>- Set 4: 1 minute

4×20 Cable Oblique Bends

Workout 19: Chest and Shoulders

4 × 10 Walking Push-Ups

Medicine Ball Circles

> 3 Sets
>
> - Set 1: 12 Reps
>
> - Set 2: 15 Reps
>
> - Set 3: 20 Reps

Incline Push-Ups

> 4 Sets
>
> - Set 1: 12 Reps
>
> - Set 2: 15 Reps
>
> - Set 3: 15 Reps
>
> - Set 4: 20 Reps

2 × 20 Decline Push-Ups

3 × 15 Rear Laterals

Workout 20: Arms, Abs, Lower Back/Hips

Cable Hammer Curls

> 4 Sets
>
> - Set 1: 12 Reps
>
> - Set 2: 15 Reps
>
> - Set 3: 15 Reps
>
> - Set 4: 20 Reps

Medicine Ball Arm Curls

> 3 Sets
>
> - Set 1: 12 Reps
>
> - Set 2: 15 Reps
>
> - Set 3: 15 Reps

4 × 20 Triceps Dips

3 × 15 Triceps Cable Extensions

Ball Crunches

> 4 Sets
>
> - Set 1: 15 Reps
>
> - Set 2: 20 Reps
>
> - Set 3: 20 Reps
>
> - Set 4: 25 Reps

3 × 15 Hip Draws

Hip Twists

> 3 Sets
>
> - Set 1: 8 Reps
>
> - Set 2: 10 Reps
>
> - Set 3: 12 Reps

Workout 21: Legs

Lunges

> 4 Sets
>
> - Set 1: 15 Reps
>
> - Set 2: 15 Reps
>
> - Set 3: 20 Reps
>
> - Set 4: 20 Reps

3 × 15 Medicine Ball Squat-Presses

Knee Drops

> 3 Sets
>
> - Set 1: 18 Reps
>
> - Set 2: 20 Reps
>
> - Set 3: 20 Reps

3 × 1-minute Squat Holds

4 × 15 Hamstring Lifts

Workout 22: Core

2 × 25 Standard Crunches

2 × 20 Rotating Crunches

2 × 15 Leg Lifts

2 × 10 V-Ups

1 × 1-minute Flat Planks

1 × 1-minute Tall Planks

1 × 1-minute Side Planks

Arm Lifts

      3 Sets

      - Set 1: 10 Reps

      - Set 2: 10 Reps

      - Set 3: 12 Reps

2 × 8 Bridges

Workout 23: Chest and Shoulders

4 × 15 Medicine Ball Circles

Medicine Ball Overhead Presses

      4 Sets

       - Set 1: 15 Reps

       - Set 2: 20 Reps

       - Set 3: 25 Reps

       - Set 4: 25 Reps

3 × 10 Walking Push-Ups

Diamond Push-Ups

      3 Sets

       - Set 1: 10 Reps

       - Set 2: 10 Reps

       - Set 3: 12 Reps

4 × 15 Dip Push-Ups

4 × 20 Push-Ups

Workout 24: Arms and Back

Table Pulls

> 4 Sets
>
> - Set 1: 8 Reps
>
> - Set 2: 10 Reps
>
> - Set 3: 12 Reps
>
> - Set 4: 12 Reps

4 × 15 Exercise Ball Back Exercises

Cable Column Rows

> 4 Sets
>
> - Set 1: 15 Reps
>
> - Set 2: 15 Reps
>
> - Set 3: 20 Reps
>
> - Set 4: 20 Reps

5 × 15 Cable Curls

Triceps Dips

> 5 Sets
>
> - Set 1: 12 Reps
>
> - Set 2: 12 Reps
>
> - Set 3: 15 Reps
>
> - Set 4: 15 Reps
>
> - Set 5: 15 Reps

Triceps Cable Extensions

> 3 Sets
>
> - Set 1: 12 Reps
>
> - Set 2: 15 Reps
>
> - Set 3: 15 Reps

Workout 25: Lower Body

3 × 12 Hamstring Leans

One-Leg Chair Dips

    4 Sets

    - Set 1: 10 Reps

    - Set 2: 10 Reps

    - Set 3: 12 Reps

    - Set 4: 12 Reps

Elevated Bridges

    3 Sets

    - Set 1: 15 Reps

    - Set 2: 15 Reps

    - Set 3: 20 Reps

Squats

    4 Sets

    - Set 1: 18 Reps

    - Set 2: 20 Reps

    - Set 3: 25 Reps

    - Set 4: 25 Reps

2 × 10 Squat Jumps

Drop Sets, Supersets, Partials,and Failure

Now that you have 25 workouts and myriad movement practice under your belt, it's time to get acquainted with a few more techniques to further advance your training. These techniques are called *drop sets*, *supersets*, *partials*, and *failure*. Here's what's involved:

Drop Sets: A drop set simply involves immediately switching to a lighter weight once you can no longer complete another rep of one exercise, or after completing a given number of reps.

For example, if you're doing medicine ball presses with a 15-pound medicine ball and, after 13 reps, you can't complete another full rep, you can drop the 15-pound medicine ball, pick up a 10-pound medicine ball, and do two more reps to complete the planned 15 reps.

Similarly, if you're doing medicine ball presses with a 15-pound medicine ball and complete 10 reps, you can exchange the 15-pound medicine ball for a lighter one and complete 10 more reps.

Superset: A superset is doing two or more exercises back-to-back without a break. For example, you might do 15 reps of squats and then immediately begin doing lunges for three lengths of the room.

Partials: Partials are a method of fully exhausting a muscle. You complete as many full reps of an exercise as possible and, when you can no longer do anymore, you do as many three-quarter, then half, then quarter-reps as possible. Those reps that are not full range of motion are called partials.

Failure: To go to failure is to do an exercise until you simply can't do it anymore.

Workout 26: Chest

Two-Hand Medicine Ball Push-Ups

    4 Sets

    - Set 1: 10 Reps

    - Set 2: 10 Reps

    - Set 3: 12 Reps

    - Set 4: 12 Reps

Plyometric Push-Ups

    3 Sets

    - Set 1: 5 Reps

    - Set 2: 7 Reps

    - Set 3: 8 Reps

4×20 Cable Chest Presses

2×15 Cable Post Flies

Workout 27: Arms

Cable Curls

    3 Sets

    - Set 1: 12 Reps

    - Set 2: 15 Reps

    - Set 3: 15 Reps

1 × Failure Cable Curls

Medicine Ball Triceps Extensions

    4 Sets

    - Set 1: 12 Reps

    - Set 2: 15 Reps

    - Set 3: 20 Reps

    - Set 4: 20 Reps

1 × Failure Medicine Ball Triceps Extensions

3 × 15 Triceps Dips

3 × 20 Cable Hammer Curls

Workout 28: Lower Body

1 × 30-second Squat Hold

   Superset into 20 Squats

1 × 1-minute Squat Hold

   Superset into 15 Squats

1 × 90-second Squat Hold

   Superset into 10 Squats

Lunges

   3 Sets

   - Set 1: 20 Reps

   - Set 2: 25 Reps

   - Set 3: 25 Reps

3 × 15 One-Leg Elevated Bridges

4 × Failure One-Leg Calf Raises

Workout 29: Shoulders and Back

Shoulder Push-Ups

>   4 Sets
>
>   - Set 1: 10 Reps
>
>   - Set 2: 12 Reps
>
>   - Set 3: 15 Reps
>
>   - Set 4: 15 Reps

3 × Failure Side Laterals

3 × Failure Cable Overhead Presses

Rear Laterals

>   3 Sets
>
>   - Set 1: 15 Reps
>
>   - Set 2: 18 Reps
>
>   - Set 3: 20 Reps

4 × 12 Table Pulls

Cable Column Rows

>   4 Sets
>
>   - Set 1: 15 Reps
>
>   - Set 2: 18 Reps
>
>   - Set 3: 20 Reps
>
>   - Set 4: 20 Reps

3 × Failure Lying Arm Raises: Side

Workout 30: Core

Standard Crunches

>   3 Sets
>
>   - Set 1: 20 Reps
>
>   - Set 2: 25 Reps
>
>   - Set 3: 30 Reps

Single-Knee Bends

>   4 Sets
>
>   - Set 1: 10 Reps
>
>   - Set 2: 12 Reps
>
>   - Set 3: 15 Reps
>
>   - Set 4: 18 Reps

2 sets of Ball Crunches, until you've done five partials (five crunches at the end of the set where you can't do a full crunch, but you still go as far as you can).

3 × Failure Push-Up Walk-Outs

4 × 15 Leg Sways

Workout 31: Chest & Arms

2 × 20 Alternating Leg Raise Push-Ups

2 × 20 Incline Push-Ups

2 × Failure Decline Push-Ups

2 × 25 Cable Chest Presses

2 sets of Cable Chest Flies, until you've done five partials

Cable Hammer Curls

 3 Sets

 - Set 1: 15 Reps

 - Set 2: 18 Reps

 - Set 3: 20 Reps

Triceps Dips

 3 Sets

 - Set 1: 15 Reps

 - Set 2: 18 Reps

 - Set 3: 20 Reps

2 × Failure Cable Curls

2 × Failure Triceps Dips

Workout 32: Legs

3 × 15 Squat Jumps

Knee Drops

   4 Sets

   - Set 1: 15 Reps

   - Set 2: 20 Reps

   - Set 3: 20 Reps

   - Set 4: 25 Reps

2 × 8 One-Leg Chair Squats

2 × Failure Leaning Squats

Exercise Ball Hamstring Curls

   3 Sets

   - Set 1: 15 Reps

   - Set 2: 15 Reps

   - Set 3: 20 Reps

Workout 33: Shoulders & Back

Cable Overhead Presses

    5 Sets

    - Set 1: 12 Reps

    - Set 2: 15 Reps

    - Set 3: 20 Reps

    - Set 4: 20 Reps

    - Set 5: 25 Reps

2 sets of Front Lateral Raises until seven partials

2 sets of Rear Lateral Raises until seven partials

Medicine Ball Circles

    3 Sets

    - Set 1: 15 Reps

    - Set 2: 20 Reps

    - Set 3: 20 Reps

4×25 Medicine Ball Rows

$2 \times$ Failure Table Pulls

$3 \times$ Failure Cable Column Rows

Workout 34: Core

Elevated Side Planks

      3 Sets

      - Set 1: 1 minute

      - Set 2: 1 minute

      - Set 3: 90 seconds

1 × Failure Flat Plank

3 × 15 Medicine Ball Turns

Hip Lifts

      3 Sets

      - Set 1: 15 Reps

      - Set 2: 20 Reps

      - Set 3: 20 Reps

2 × Failure Ball Crunches

Workout 35: Chest & Arms

Cable Chest Presses

> 4 Sets
>
> - Set 1: 15 Reps
>
> - Set 2: 20 Reps
>
> - Set 3: 20 Reps
>
> - Set 4: 25 Reps

3 × Failure Push-Ups

3 × Failure Dip Push-Ups

2 × 15 One-Hand Medicine Ball Push-Ups

3 × Failure Cable Curls

2 × Failure Cable Hammer Curls

3 sets of Triceps Dips until seven partials

Cardio Circuits

These cardio routines are sure to get you sweating in short order and melt the fat off your body. Some are brief but require high intensity, while others involve less effort but last longer. Keep your workouts mixed up and you'll not only have more fun while you train, but you'll also keep your body working efficiently and always guessing—a surefire recipe for success.

Use these routines to get you going and, once you're comfortable, feel free to create your own using a mixture of the elements contained here and any others you find useful. Tailor them to your needs and your enjoyment, and you'll quickly create a healthy habit for life.

As you go through these cardio workouts, keep in mind that they, like the training workouts, are built in order of increasing difficulty. Some may find the first few routines too easy, while others will find them a perfect place to start. Feel free to skip ahead if necessary; likewise, feel free to stick to the first few routines until you're conditioned enough to move forward. Also, unless otherwise noted, there is no rest between exercises. You are to switch right from one into the other and only break when indicated in the routine. If no break or repeat is indicated, that is the end of the routine.

Cardio Routine 1

1 minute: Jog in Place

30 seconds: Butt Kicking

Repeat three times, break for one minute, and repeat three more times.

Cardio Routine 2

1 minute: Jog in Place

30 seconds: High Knees

30 seconds: Butt Kicking

Repeat three times, break for one minute, and repeat three more times.

Cardio Routine 3

1 minute: Jumping Jacks

30 seconds: High Knees

30 seconds: Butt Kicking

Repeat three times, break for one minute, and repeat three more times.

Cardio Routine 4

1 minute: Jog in Place

1 minute: Jumping Jacks

1 minute: High Knees

Repeat four times.

Cardio Routine 5

1 minute: Jumping Jacks

1 minute: High Knees

1 minute: Butt Kicking

1 minute: Toe Kicks

Repeat three times, break for 30 seconds, and repeat two more times.

Cardio Routine 6

1 minute: Star Picker

1 minute: High Knees

1 minute: Jumping Jacks

Repeat three times, break for one minute, and repeat three more times.

Cardio Routine 7

2 minutes: Jog in Place

1 minute: Dual Squats

2 minutes: Jumping Jacks

Repeat three times.

Cardio Routine 8

1 minute: Side Steps

1 minute: Long Leaps

1 minute: Mountain Climbers

2 minutes: Jog in Place

Repeat twice, break for thirty seconds, and repeat twice more.

Cardio Routine 9

1 minute: Ski Jumps

1 minute: Long Leaps

1 minute: Star Picker

1 minute: High Knees

1 minute: Butt Kicking, as fast as possible

Break for one minute, repeat, break for one minute, and repeat once more.

Cardio Routine 10

2 minutes: Jumping Jacks

30 seconds: Jog in Place, feet moving as fast as possible

30 seconds: Break

Repeat three times.

Cardio Routine 11

1 minute: Push-Up U-Jumps

1 minute: Knee Jumps

1 minute: Break

Repeat five times.

Cardio Routine 12

1 minute: Hop Jumps

1 minute: Dual Squats

30 seconds: Break

Repeat five times.

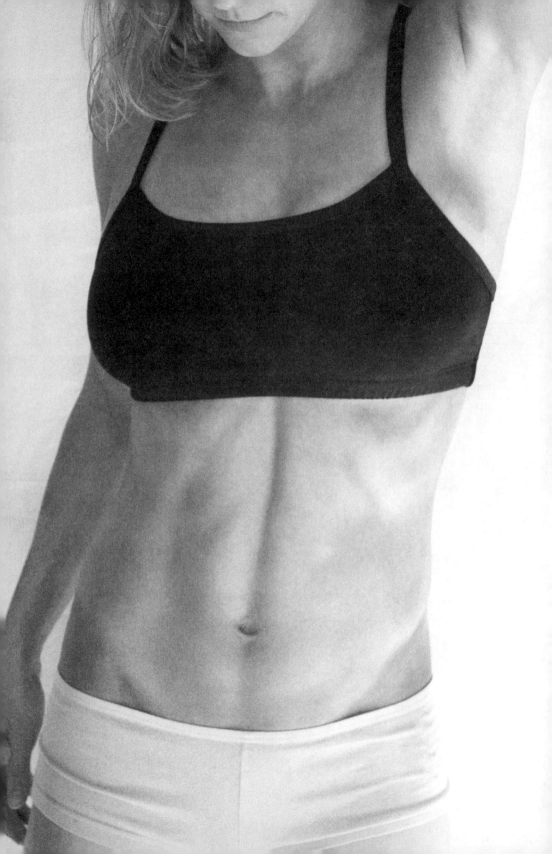

9

Beyond the Workout: After-Training Tips

You already know that your workout and the foods that you use to fuel your body are the most important parts of getting the toned, fit body that you seek. But there are plenty of other key things to think about that don't involve training. You shouldn't ignore the value of rest, but on the flip side, there are plenty of fancy supplement ads you *should* ignore.

Rest and Recovery

Despite the way it may seem, you don't add muscle during training. You may be burning some calories and getting rid of a little body fat, but even those processes mostly occur when you aren't working out. Instead, it happens when you're resting. To get the most out of your training you need to pay close attention to what you're doing during the 23 or so hours a day you're not exercising.

When You Grow: The True Value of Sleep

You burn fat and add muscle when you sleep. Think of your body changing in the same way you would think of baking a cake. You put all of the ingredients and hard work in on the counter, outside of the oven, and only after all the effort has been expended can you place it in the oven and let it do its thing. Your body works quite a bit on that same principle. The work you do during the day (or night, depending on your schedule) sets you up for the changes that will be made, good or bad. If you're eating properly and training right, your body will repair muscle tissue, add muscle tissue, and burn fat all day, and particularly while you sleep. When it can focus on just getting rid of unwanted fat and building new strong, lean tissue, your body is very happy. Your job is to give it that opportunity.

More and more studies show the vast benefits of proper sleep. And it isn't just physical; research on the mental component of sleep has found that it's more difficult to learn new information after just one night of disturbed sleep. Additionally, people who fail to get enough sleep night after night are at a much higher risk of chronic diseases like diabetes, high blood pressure, and heart disease.

Sleep is a wonderful thing for the body in more ways than you could ever imagine. So if you're not getting *at least* six hours of sleep a night, you're robbing yourself of progress. In the ideal world, eight hours of sleep would be best, but in an increasingly hectic world, there are a few things we have to be proud of if we can even hit the bare minimum. Sleep is often one of those things. No matter what kind of planning it takes, rearrange your schedule to allow for adequate sleep.

The Risk of Overtraining

When you don't sleep, you're continuing to run your body in a compromised state. And when you continually keep up a level of activity that your body can't support because it's not getting enough recovery time, you end up with a reduced immune system and run the serious risk of overtraining. You can make yourself sick, sure, but you can also create a state where the body burns muscle instead of fat to function, which will undo all of the hard work you've put in.

Overtraining can also be called under-recovering, because the body can do quite well with heavy training as long as it's adequately repaid for its efforts. But you must make sure you match your exercise volume with the amount of recovery you get. Otherwise, it's all for naught.

Speaking of Supplements

One way to increase recovery ability is through the use of dietary and nutritional supplements. You can't miss them; they're everywhere. From superstores set up strictly for their display and sale to the dedicated aisles you see in grocery stores, there are hundreds—no, thousands—of types of supplements available today. The key is to know which are worth your money, which are like throwing money away, and—worst of all—which can be harmful.

Debunking Supplement Ads

It doesn't matter if you're reading *Muscular Development* or *Mom's Monthly*, you're going to see advertisements in magazines for a variety of supplements. Some promise more energy, others promise increased fat loss, and still others promise "600% more muscle" or that they're "better than steroids."

When it comes to supplements, if a claim sounds too good to be true, it is. No legal supplement is going to work like a steroid, and if it did, it wouldn't be on the market. Steroids are hormonal drugs that carry the risk of adverse side effects and are strongly regulated. While there are steroid precursors (hormone metabolites that have to be converted in the liver to its active steroidal form) on the market that are considered to be the next big thing, you should avoid them. They lack long-term studies and are potentially dangerous.

Supplements are *exactly* what they say they are: supplemental. They can't, and won't, do the hard work for you. Perhaps they'll help burn a few extra calories, but they won't take pounds of fat off your belly. They may help you recover more quickly, but not to the point you can skip out on an hour of sleep. They may blunt your appetite, but you still have to choose healthy foods when you do eat.

Supplements Facts

Nutritional supplements are a multi-billion dollar industry in large part because they charge notoriously high mark-ups on their products. You may think that because a fat burner costs $39.95, it has high-quality ingredients, but often, this isn't the case. Many supplements that sell in the $20 to $40 range cost only $2 to $4 a bottle to make, which translates into serious profits for the manufacturer. The moral of this story: more expensive doesn't mean better. Use your gut and your brain and do your research. If it sounds too good to be true, it is. If they're making an outrageous claim, it doesn't take more than a quick search on Bing or Google to find out if it's true. More often than not, there are other people who made the unfortunate mistake of buying whatever it is you're reading about, and their review will tell you all you need to know.

Even in high-quality supplements, you should be aware that your body might not be using—or even getting—everything that's on the label. Sometimes this is because the ingredient amounts listed on the bottle are incorrect, overestimated, or misrepresented. However, the major problem is that your body often can't absorb such a large amount of a particular ingredient at once, and the extra passes through your body without being used. There are also other factors affecting what your body can use, such as your level of hydration, other foods you've eaten, and what supplements you're taking with each other (certain minerals fight for absorption in the body).

So while a multivitamin may be a valuable addition to your daily program, don't think that it includes all of the nutrients you need in a day. You still need a balanced diet to ensure your body gets everything it needs.

When it comes to fat burners, or thermogenics as they're often called, don't expect them to do the proverbial heavy lifting for you. While they may increase your metabolism, we're talking only perhaps a couple dozen calories a day. And when you realize that a pound of fat equates to 3,500 excess calories, it's a long, long road ahead if you're counting on a supplement to burn off all that fat.

The real benefit to fat burners and things like energy drinks are that they may help you feel better and more enthused to work out, which can help you train longer and harder. In the end, this may result in more fat loss, but the direct correlation between supplements and burning calories is extremely tenuous.

Supplements That Work

I don't want you to think that supplements are a total waste of your hard-earned money. There are plenty of supplements that work and that you might find worth buying.

Glucosamine/chondroitin/MSM for joint pain. If you have joint pain, a very common ailment in adults, you might find a glucosamine/chondroitin/MSM supplement useful. Glucosamine helps make the minerals that help comprise cartilage. Chondroitin is another component in cartilage and works even better when combined with glucosamine. The final ingredient, methylsulfonylmethane (MSM), is a sulfur compound that helps repair connective tissues and reduces inflammation. Many people have reported great results with this; however, it should be noted that it isn't for people with shellfish allergies.

Creatine to increase strength and muscle mass. Creatine is one of the most popular and beneficial supplements on the market and is effective for both men and women. Study after study shows that creatine use increases strength and fat-free mass in users and is safe and effective for healthy adults. The most effective form of this supplement is plain monohydrate powder that can be mixed into your drink of choice. Don't be fooled into paying more for proprietary blends of creatine. Stick with the basic form, which is cheap and has been proven effective.

Coenzyme Q-10 for a host of benefits. Coenzyme Q-10 has been used over time to help numerous conditions, including congestive heart failure, Huntington's disease, Parkinson's disease, hypertension, and migraines. It occurs naturally in foods such as beef and fish, but increased doses from supplements are useful as well.

Vitamin D for overall health. A very low percentage of the country gets adequate vitamin D from sunshine. With the proliferation of reasons people stay indoors these days, a supplement is often the best bet way to catch up on our bodily requirements. Vitamin D plays a role in everything from cell growth to immune function to reducing inflammation. Vitamin D is cheap, easy to find, and one of the more important supplements you can buy.

Protein Shakes: Casein, Soy, and Whey

Without a doubt, one of the most beneficial—and likely *the* most effective supplement on the market today—is protein powder.

Protein does a litany of good for the body. It can help blunt hunger, repair muscle tissue, help the body burn fat more effectively, assist in keeping blood sugar regulated in the body as well as many more great deeds. As you can see, the benefits of protein are numerous, and having a quick, convenient, and tasty method of increasing your intake is a welcome advance of science.

Protein supplements tend to be divided into three types based on their composition and structure. Here's an overview:

Casein protein: The body absorbs casein protein slowly, which is useful prior to a period of time when you'll be going without food. This includes sleep, though the jury is out on whether or not casein is more effective than other types of protein as far as preventing muscle breakdown and preventing the body from turning to a catabolic (muscle eating) state. It seems to provide people with a more enduring sense of satiety, which can help prevent overeating.

Soy protein: This is a great option for vegans who can't use milk-based products (casein and whey are both derived from milk). Soy protein is high in glutamine (which helps reduce muscle breakdown) and other amino acids and has been shown in some studies to improve lipid profiles (cholesterol, a risk panel for coronary disease) and even kidney function.

Whey protein: In general, whey is considered the ultimate in muscle-building protein supplementation. It tends to be the cheapest and is absorbed by the body the most quickly. This makes it ideal first thing in the morning, when your body is begging for nutrition, or after a workout, when your body has an increased ability to absorb protein. One key benefit of whey protein for people who want to get toned is that it boosts the levels of hunger-stopping hormones in the body (such as cholecystokinin) that help us eat less later on. But whey protein isn't the only beneficial form of protein.

Two other relatively common protein powders on the market are made from eggs and rices, but they are not nearly as popular and don't offer any advantages over casein, soy, and whey protein.

Concentrates vs. Isolates

When you look at ingredients on a protein supplement bottle, the protein will most often either be listed in concentrate or isolate form. The most common form is concentrate, but the better version is isolate. Think of it like juice; from concentrate, or fresh squeezed. The concentrate form has fillers, such as fats and carbohydrates, and often they are high in cholesterol. The isolates are processed to remove lactose and fats and tend to be significantly higher in total protein by volume compared to concentrates.

If it fits your budget, the isolate version is superior, tastes better, and is made with far fewer fats and carbohydrates.

Timing

You should have a protein shake immediately after each workout to help kick-start the recovery and growth process of your workout. You can also, of course, have a protein shake anytime you're in need of a quick, highly nutritious, muscle-building meal. They travel well and are as quick as anything else you could possibly eat (or, rather, drink!).

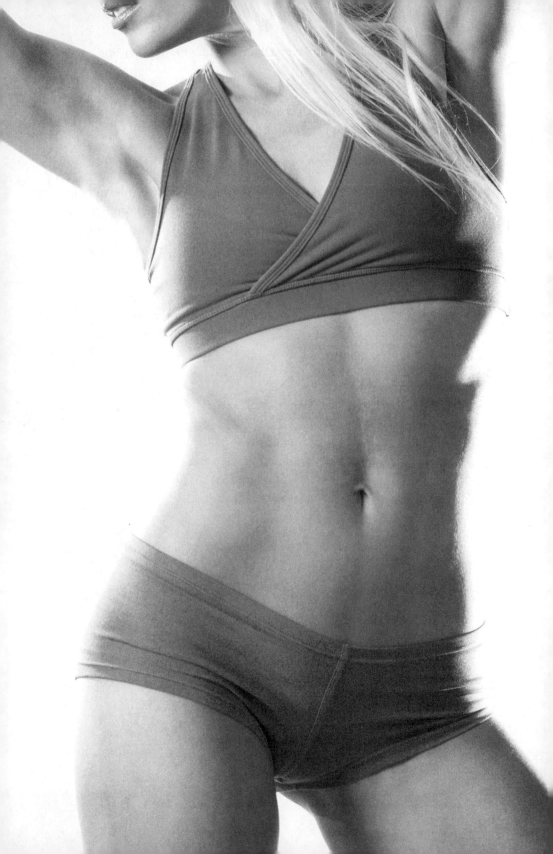

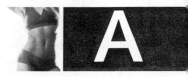

Glossary

aerobic   With the presence of oxygen. In fitness, refers to long-duration, sustainable cardiovascular exercise.

amino acid   The building blocks from which proteins are made.

anaerobic   Without the use of oxygen; for fitness purposes, refers to high-intensity, short-duration exercise.

aspartame   Artificial sweetener marketed as "Equal."

bromelain   An element with anti-inflammatory properties.

casein   A type of protein derived from milk that is slower to digest in the human body than whey protein.

Coenzyme Q10 (Co Q-10)   A popular nutritional supplement shown to improve cardiovascular health; also known as *Ubiquinone*.

cortisol   Stress hormone that encourages the likelihood of calories being stored as fat.

creatine   An amino acid that encourages the body to store extra energy in muscles.

drop set   A continuous set of exercises in which the weight of an exercise is lowered after the first set with the goal of doing more repetitions.

forced rep   A training repetition that can't be completed alone using strict form by the person exercising; it is often conducted with the help of a partner or body movement.

gluten   A substance found in wheat and other grains that is responsible for texture of dough; many people have allergies to gluten.

glycemic index   A ranking system for carbohydrates that refers to the speed at which they are converted into glucose and their effect on blood-sugar levels.

HDL cholesterol   High-density lipoprotein, sometimes called the "good cholesterol."

hydrogenated oil   *See* trans fat

LDL cholesterol   Low-density lipoprotein; often referred to as the "bad cholesterol."

metabolism   The total energy burned by the body to maintain homeostasis and normal function.

modified food starch   A food starch that has been modified in some way; manufacturers are not required to describe the type of modification.

multi-grain   A combination of grains, most often refined, put together to make a particular food.

negative calorie   Food myth referring to foods that supposedly burn more calories during digestion than they contain.

organic   Foods made without chemicals and most other man-made fertilizers and insecticides.

overtraining   A state in which the body can not recover to baseline hormone and lactate levels due to an increase in training stress.

partial rep   Partial repetitions done at the end of a set after the person exercising can no longer complete full range-of-motion repetitions.

partially hydrogenated oil   *See* trans fat

recovery   The process of the body resting and receiving adequate nutrition and sleep to allow for the repair and growth of muscle fibers.

sea salt   A type of salt containing trace minerals.

serving size   The suggested portion size of a food; does not usually refer to all of the contents inside a container.

split   In fitness, a training routine that defines specific exercise and rest days.

static   Exercises that are done by holding one position; not moving.

sucralose   Artificial sweetener marketed as "Splenda."

superset   Two exercises targeting the same muscle or muscle group(s) conducted back-to-back without pausing for rest in between.

trans fat   A polyunsaturated fatty acid created by the process of hydrogenation that are very difficult for the body to process.

turmeric   A spice with known anti-inflammatory properties.

volume   In fitness, the total sum of training.

warm-up   A process of performing easy, slow motions to prepare the muscles for more intense exercises to follow.

whey   A milk-derived protein popular among workout enthusiasts for the speed at which it digests in the body, thus allowing for the uptake of amino acids more quickly. Most often used immediately post-exercise.

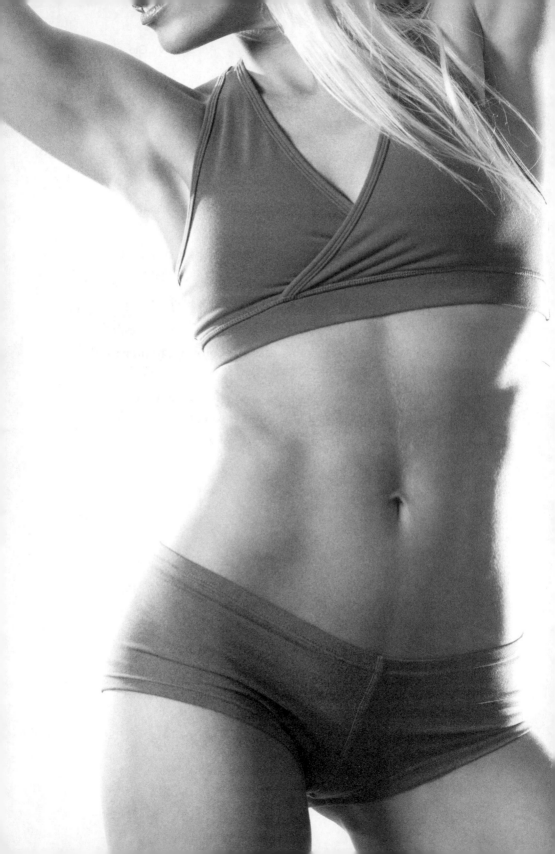

Food for You: Nutritious Recipes

Undoubtedly you already have plenty of healthy foods you enjoy making, but it always helps to spice up your diet with new, healthful recipes. Adding new nutritious meals to your gym-free and toned lifestyle helps keep you from going back to high-calorie, low-nutrient staples that you might have relied on in the past for a quick meal or a snack.

From recipes for protein shakes to steaks to tofu, you can add the foods in this appendix to your eating schedule to help you achieve your training goals.

Liquid Nutrition: Shakes and Smoothies

Healthy OJ

Create your own healthy, creamy orange shake.

Yield:	Prep time:	Cook time:	Serving size:
1 shake	5 minutes	N/A	8 oz.

Each serving has:
220 calories
1 g fat
30 g carbohydrates
25 g protein

1 serving vanilla whey protein   1 cup orange juice

1. Place vanilla whey protein and orange juice in blender or shaker cup and blend/shake until desired consistency is reached.

Iced Greek Coffee

This is a sweet coffee treat without the calories of the big chain coffeeshop drinks.

Yield:	Prep time:	Cook time:	Serving size:
1 coffee	5 minutes	N/A	1 cup

Each serving has:
60 calories
1 g fat
10 g carbohydrates
3 g protein

2 tsp. house blend (or choice) instant coffee	2-4 ice cubes
1 tsp. sugar	$\frac{1}{4}$ cup water
	$\frac{1}{3}$ cup fat-free milk

1. Combine instant coffee, sugar, ice cubs, and water in thermos or pitcher. Cover and shake until mixture is frothy.

2. Stir in milk.

Weight Gainer Pumpkin Shake

When you're looking to put on weight, you need to enjoy it because eating constantly can get tedious. Try this October-inspired shake for quick, nutritious calories.

Yield:	Prep time:	Cook time:	Serving size:
1 shake	5 minutes	N/A	2½ cups

Each serving has:
600 calories
10 g fat
75 g carbohydrates
50 g protein

2 cups vanilla almond milk	½ cup canned pumpkin pie mix
50 g whey protein powder	1 tsp. ground cinnamon

1. Combine vanilla almond milk, whey protein powder, canned pumpkin pie mix, and cinnamon in blender and mix to desired consistency.

Blueberry Smoothie

A sweet smoothie with light fruit flavor thanks to a combination of almond milk and blueberries; this is sure to hit the spot.

Yield:	Prep time:	Cook time:	Serving size:
1 smoothie	5 minutes	N/A	2½ cups

Each serving has:
380 calories
21 g fat
37 g carbohydrates
31 g protein

⅓ cup low-fat cottage cheese	1 cup blueberries
1 serving whey protein	2 TB. walnuts
1 cup almond milk	2 TB. flaxseed meal

1. Combine cottage cheese, whey protein, almond milk, blueberries, walnuts, and flaxseed meal in blender and mix to desired consistency.

Anytime Smoothie

Some foods are better enjoyed at certain times of the day, but this smoothie is sweet and ready whenever you are.

Yield:	Prep time:	Cook time:	Serving size:
1 smoothie	5 minutes	N/A	2 cups

Each serving has:
300 calories
5 g fat
60 g carbohydrates
8 g protein

1 cup mixed berries	$\frac{1}{2}$ cup apple juice
$\frac{1}{2}$ large banana	$\frac{1}{4}$ cup silken tofu

1. Combine berries, banana, apple juice, and tofu in blender and mix to desired consistency.

Apricot Smoothie

Adding apricots to your smoothie gives an underappreciated fruit new life and your diet new variety.

Yield:	Prep time:	Cook time:	Serving size:
1 smoothie	5 minutes	N/A	2 cups

Each serving has:
200 calories
0 g fat
50 g carbohydrates
8 g protein

1 cup apricots (fresh or dry), halved   3 TB. sugar
1 cup fat-free vanilla yogurt   6 ice cubes

1. Combine apricots, yogurt, sugar, and ice cubs in blender and blend until frothy.

Banana Shake

Bananas are an old-time favorite; here is a new way to enjoy them.

Yield:	Prep time:	Cook time:	Serving size:
1 shake	5 minutes	N/A	2 cups

Each serving has:
160 calories
3 g fat
27 g carbohydrates
8 g protein

1 cup 1 percent milk

½ cup fat-free vanilla yogurt

1 banana

¼ tsp. vanilla extract

1. Combine milk, yogurt, banana, and vanilla extract in blender and mix to desired consistency.

Soy Smoothie

Whether you eat soy out of principle or just want to try something new, this smoothie is a healthy twist to your daily drinks.

Yield:	Prep time:	Cook time:	Serving size:
1 smoothie	5 minutes	N/A	$1\frac{1}{2}$ cups

Each serving has:
350 calories
10 g fat
55 g carbohydrates
20 g protein

1 banana

$\frac{1}{2}$ cup silken tofu

$\frac{1}{2}$ cup soymilk

2 TB. cocoa powder

1 TB. honey

1. Combine banana, tofu, soymilk, cocoa powder, and honey in blender and mix to desired consistency.

Five-Minute Meals

Tuna-Wheat Crumble

For some, the taste of tuna can be a little overpowering. By adding some crumbled crackers, you mellow the flavor and create a new meal.

Yield:	Prep time:	Cook time:	Serving size:
1 serving	3 minutes	N/A	1 can

Each serving has:
250 calories
12 g fat
15 g carbohydrates
30 g protein

1 5-oz. can tuna (in water)	2 TB. relish
2 TB. mayonnaise made with olive oil	10 whole-wheat crackers, crumbled

1. Drain tuna and place in bowl.

2. Using a fork, mix in mayonnaise, relish, and cracker crumbles.

Raisin-Pecan Oatmeal

Oatmeal doesn't have to be boring, and this sweet, fruit-infused meal proves it.

Yield:	Prep time:	Cook time:	Serving size:
1 bowl	10 minutes	Varies	$\frac{1}{3}$ cup

Each serving has:
300 calories
10 g fat
33 g carbohydrates
7 g protein

$\frac{1}{3}$ cup rolled oats	$\frac{1}{4}$ tsp. ground nutmeg
1 TB. butter	$\frac{1}{4}$ tsp. ground cinnamon
1 TB. raisins	1 tsp. chopped pecans

1. Prepare oatmeal per manufacturer directions.

2. Add butter, raisins, nutmeg, cinnamon, and pecans to oatmeal and stir.

Pina-Colada-Inspired Yogurt

Yogurt can get mundane, so try sprucing it up with a drink favorite.

Yield:	Prep time:	Cook time:	Serving size:
1 serving	2 minutes	N/A	$\frac{1}{3}$ cup

Each serving has:
150 calories
3 g fat
25 g carbohydrates
9 g protein

$\frac{1}{3}$ cup low-fat vanilla yogurt   1 TB. toasted coconut
$\frac{1}{2}$ cup crushed pineapple, drained

1. Combine yogurt and pineapple and top with coconut.

Strawberry Chia Yogurt

Adding chia to your yogurt offers a slightly toasted flavor with an amazing omega-3 punch.

Yield:	Prep time:	Cook time:	Serving size:
1 serving	2 minutes	N/A	¾ cup

Each serving has:
170 calories
5 g fat
23 g carbohydrates
11 g protein

¾ cup fat-free strawberry yogurt   1 TB. chia seeds

1. Combine yogurt and chia and mix well.

Cottage Cheese Breakfast Treat

Cottage cheese on its own doesn't offer much flavor, but adding pineapple or peaches sweetens the deal.

Yield:	Prep time:	Cook time:	Serving size:
1 serving	2 minutes	N/A	1 cup

Each serving has:
300 calories
10 g fat
30 g carbohydrates
20 g protein

1 cup 2 percent milkfat cottage cheese

1 cup pineapple tidbits or cubed peaches

2 tsp. toasted wheat germ

1. Mix cottage cheese and pineapple or peaches in a bowl and top with wheat germ.

Fruity Muesli

Like plain oatmeal, Muesli can be a bit bland, so adding fruit will make it a surefire go-to during your day.

Yield:	Prep time:	Cook time:	Serving size:
1 serving	3 minutes	N/A	$\frac{1}{2}$ cup

Each serving has:
300 calories
5 g fat
60 g carbohydrates
15 g protein

$\frac{1}{2}$ cup low-fat plain yogurt

$\frac{1}{2}$ cup blueberries

$\frac{1}{4}$ cup diced apple

$\frac{1}{4}$ cup diced banana

1 tsp. honey

$\frac{1}{4}$ cup unsweetened muesli

1. Combine yogurt, blueberries, apple, banana, honey, and muesli in bowl.

Microwave Scramble

Eggs don't have to take much time nor do they have to make a mess—try them in the microwave.

Yield:	Prep time:	Cook time:	Serving size:
1 serving	5 minutes	$1\frac{1}{2}$ minutes	1 cup

Each serving has:
180 calories
15 g fat
4 g carbohydrates
18 g protein

2 TB. fat-free milk	2 TB. shredded cheddar cheese
2 large eggs	Pinch of salt

1. Coat large coffee mug with nonstick spray and add milk and eggs, stirring until well mixed.

2. Microwave egg mixture for 45 seconds, stir, and then microwave another 45 seconds.

3. Sprinkle egg mixture with cheese and salt and allow to cool slightly before eating.

Salmon Sandwich

Fish doesn't always have to be eaten with a fork. Try making your own tasty fish sandwich out of delicious salmon.

Yield:	Prep time:	Cook time:	Serving size:
1 sandwich	3 minutes	N/A	1 sandwich

Each serving has:
370 calories
14 g fat
32 g carbohydrates
28 g protein

1 (4-oz.) pouch or can ready-to-eat salmon	2 slices whole-wheat or whole-grain bread
1 slice red onion, chopped	1 slice tomato
2 TB. mayonnaise made with olive oil	

1. Mix salmon, onion, and mayonnaise together until well blended.

2. Spread salmon mixture on bread, top with tomato, and serve.

Great Pre-Workout Meals

Morning Bean Melt

Beans aren't just a Mexican-themed dinner favorite anymore—they're an energy packed breakfast treat when you spice them up with salsa and cheese.

Yield:	Prep time:	Cook time:	Serving size:
1 serving	2 minutes	45 seconds	1 slice

Each serving has:
125 calories
3 g fat
20 g carbohydrates
8 g protein

1 slice whole-wheat bread	1 TB. salsa
2 TB. nonfat refried beans	1 TB. cheese of choice, grated

1. Toast whole-wheat bread in toaster.

2. Top toast with beans, salsa, and cheese, and microwave until cheese is melted and toppings are hot (about 45 seconds).

Breakfast Pita

Adding a pita to your eggs in the morning gives you a new take on the standard protein favorite.

Yield:	Prep time:	Cook time:	Serving size:
1 serving	7 minutes	5 minutes	1 pita

Each serving has:
320 calories
24 g fat
19 g carbohydrates
23 g protein

$\frac{1}{4}$ cup diced onion	1 egg white
$\frac{1}{4}$ cup diced green bell pepper	$\frac{1}{4}$ cup feta cheese, crumbled
2 whole eggs	1 whole-wheat pita

1. Place onion and green pepper in nonstick pan and sauté for two minutes.

2. Add eggs and egg white to vegetables and scramble.

3. Just before eggs are done, add cheese and allow to melt.

4. Place in pita and enjoy.

Multi-Grain Waffles

Just because you're eating healthy doesn't mean you can't have waffles any longer; try this multi-grain mix for a fluffy, tasty breakfast.

Yield:	Prep time:	Cook time:	Serving size:
8 servings	15 minutes	4-5 minutes	2 waffles

Each serving has:
200 calories
5 g fat
25 g carbohydrates
7 g protein

2 cups buttermilk

½ cup rolled oats

⅔ cup all-purpose flour

⅔ cup whole-wheat flour

¼ cup toasted wheat germ

1½ tsp. baking powder

¼ tsp. salt

1 tsp. ground cinnamon

½ tsp. baking soda

2 eggs, beaten

1 TB. canola oil

2 tsp. vanilla extract

¼ cup packed brown sugar

1. Combine buttermilk and oats in bowl and let stand for 10 minutes.

2. Combine all-purpose flour, wheat flour, wheat germ, baking powder, salt, cinnamon, and baking soda in separate bowl.

3. Add eggs, oil, vanilla, and brown sugar to the buttermilk mixture.

4. Combine the wet ingredients with the dry ingredients and mix, ensuring not to overmix.

5. Preheat waffle iron and cook in batches.

Apple Breakfast Oats

Adding apples gives you another opportunity to break the monotony of plain oats.

Yield:	Prep time:	Cook time:	Serving size:
1 serving	10 minutes	7 minutes	1 cup

Each serving has:
250 calories
3 g fat
50 g carbohydrates
8 g protein

1 cup quick oats	$\frac{1}{2}$ cup unsweetened applesauce
1 cup apple juice	$\frac{1}{4}$ tsp. ground cinnamon

1. Combine oats and apple juice in a saucepan and bring to a boil. Remove from heat and let stand for five minutes.

2. Add applesauce and cinnamon and stir.

Breakfast Tortillas

This is a popular home version of the breakfast wraps offered at fast-food restaurants.

Yield:	Prep time:	Cook time:	Serving size:
1 serving	8 minutes	5 minutes	2 tortillas

Each serving has:
410 calories
18 g fat
38 g carbohydrates
22 g protein

2 small corn tortillas

2 TB. cheese of choice, grated

1 TB. salsa

2 whole eggs

2 egg whites

1. Sprinkle cheese and salsa on tortillas and heat in microwave for 20 to 30 seconds.

2. Scramble eggs and egg whites in nonstick skillet over medium heat, and then divide over tortillas.

Oatmeal Cookies

Eating healthy doesn't mean giving up cookies; try this oatmeal variety to give you anytime energy.

Yield:	Prep time:	Cook time:	Serving size:
Varies	40 minutes	10-12 minutes	2 cookies

Each serving has:
80 calories
2 g fat
15 g carbohydrates
1 g protein

2 cups whole-wheat flour

2 cups quick oats

1 tsp. ground cinnamon

1 tsp. baking soda

$\frac{1}{4}$ tsp. salt

8 TB. unsalted butter, room temperature

$\frac{3}{4}$ cup sugar

1 cup brown sugar

4 egg whites

1 TB. vanilla extract

$\frac{1}{4}$ cup fat-free milk

$1\frac{1}{2}$ cups chopped nuts

1. Preheat oven to 350°F.

2. Combine flour, oats, cinnamon, baking soda, and salt.

3. Place butter in a separate bowl and mix until creamy. Add in sugars, eggs, vanilla, and milk and mix until smooth.

4. Slowly stir flour mixture into wet mixture until blended, and then stir in nuts.

5. Drop by tablespoon onto a nonstick baking pan, a few inches apart to allow for spreading. Bake 10 to 12 minutes or until cookies are lightly browned.

Breakfast Yogurt Mix

Granola gives your yogurt a chewy, sweeter flavor and more energy-laden carbohydrates.

Yield:	Prep time:	Cook time:	Serving size:
1 serving	2 minutes	N/A	1 cup

Each serving has:
300 calories
3 g fat
10 g protein
55 g carbohydrates

½ cup honey granola

1 cup blueberries

1 cup fat-free yogurt (plain or flavored)

1. Combine granola, blueberries, and yogurt and mix well.

Healthy Anytime Foods

Flank Steak with Pepper-Coffee Marinade

Coffee may seem like an odd marinade, but it makes steak tender and tasty in a whole new way.

Yield:	Prep time:	Cook time:	Serving size:
4 servings	4 hours	6-10 minutes	4 oz.

Each serving has:
250 calories
10 g fat
2 g carbohydrates
25 g protein

3 TB. brewed coffee	1 TB. brown sugar
1 TB. balsamic vinegar	$\frac{1}{2}$ tsp. salt
1 TB. extra-virgin olive oil	1 tsp. crushed black peppercorns
2 minced garlic cloves	1 lb. trimmed flank steak

1. Mix coffee, vinegar, oil, garlic, brown sugar, salt, and peppercorns in a large dish and then add steak, coating the meat in marinade. Cover and refrigerate, letting sit for up to 4 hours.

2. Set grill to high, cook steak until desired level of doneness, slice into four portions, and serve.

Egg Tortillas

This is yet another way to bring eggs into your daily meal plan, and it's suited for any time of day.

Yield:	Prep time:	Cook time:	Serving size:
1 serving	3 minutes	5 minutes	1 tortilla

Each serving has:
340 calories
22 g fat
20 g carbohydrates
20 g protein

2 whole eggs

1 egg white

$\frac{1}{4}$ cup cheddar cheese, grated

1 whole-wheat tortilla

1 TB. salsa

1. Scramble eggs and egg white in nonstick skillet with cheese.

2. When eggs are nearly done, place tortilla on top of eggs, and use steam from eggs to soften tortilla.

3. When eggs are done, place eggs in tortilla and top with salsa.

Chicken Pita Pocket

Pita's provide a new way to eat just about anything, but packing in the protein of chicken and spicing it up with chipotle is as close to perfect as you can get.

Yield:	Prep time:	Cook time:	Serving size:
1 serving	5 minutes	15 minutes	1 pita

Each serving has:
350 calories
6 g fat
19 g carbohydrates
33 g protein

1 (6-oz.) chicken breast $\frac{1}{4}$ cup chopped lettuce
1 whole-wheat pita   2 TB. chipotle sauce

1. Cook chicken breast (grilled or baked) and cut into small pieces.

2. Heat pita pocket in microwave or toaster until easily opened.

3. Place lettuce and chicken inside pita and top with chipotle sauce.

Cheesy Scramble

Cheese can be a great way to liven up protein-heavy dishes like scrambled eggs.

Yield:	Prep time:	Cook time:	Serving size:
1 serving	3 minutes	5 minutes	Entire mixture

Each serving has:
400 calories
20 g fat
4 g carbohydrates
33 g protein

3 eggs	$\frac{1}{4}$ cup 1 percent milk
3 egg whites	$\frac{1}{4}$ cup shredded low-fat cheddar cheese

1. Mix eggs, egg whites, and milk together in bowl.

2. Preheat a nonstick skillet to medium heat then add egg mixture. Stir often until eggs are scrambled and nearly done, add cheese, and then serve when cheese has melted.

Salmon & Egg Muffin

Adding salmon to this egg and muffin mix takes away the powerful fish flavor but leaves all of the protein and omega-3's intact.

Yield:	Prep time:	Cook time:	Serving size:
1 serving	5 minutes	5 minutes	1 muffin

Each serving has:
200 calories
5 g fat
23 g carbohydrates
20 g protein

$\frac{1}{2}$ tsp. extra-virgin olive oil	1 oz. smoked salmon
2 egg whites	1 slice tomato
Pinch of salt	1 whole-wheat English muffin

1. Heat oil in nonstick skillet over medium heat. Add egg whites and salt and cook until eggs are done.

2. Toast English muffin in toaster.

3. Place eggs, smoked salmon, and tomato on toasted English muffin and serve.

Royal Burger

Adding egg to your burger gives it extra protein and extra flavor!

Yield:	Prep time:	Cook time:	Serving size:
1 serving	5 minutes	6-10 minutes	1 burger

Each serving has:
560 calories
35 g fat
4 g carbohydrates
44 g protein

6 oz. 93 percent lean ground beef $\frac{1}{4}$ cup cheddar cheese, grated
$\frac{1}{4}$ cup salsa $\frac{1}{2}$ avocado, sliced
2 large eggs

1. Mix the ground beef, $\frac{1}{8}$ cup of salsa, and one egg together and form a patty.

2. On a grill or stovetop over medium heat, cook the patty to desired level doneness.

3. When patty is almost done, fry remaining egg in nonstick pan until the white is fully cooked but the yolk is soft (over easy).

4. Sprinkle shredded cheese over egg, place egg on top of beef patty, add avocado and the rest of the salsa, and serve with a fork.

Onion & Herb Italian Omelet

Omelets don't have to be plain; you can spice them up quick and easy with this onion-infused twist.

Yield:	Prep time:	Cook time:	Serving size:
1 serving	5 minutes	10 minutes	1 omelet

Each serving has:
264 calories
12 g fat
16 g carbohydrates
22 g protein

$\frac{1}{4}$ cup plus 1 tablespoon water

1 cup diced onion

1 tsp. extra-virgin olive oil

$\frac{1}{2}$ cup liquid egg substitute, such as Egg Beaters

2 tsp. chopped fresh herbs (parsley, basil), or $\frac{1}{2}$ teaspoon dried

$\frac{1}{8}$ tsp. salt

$\frac{1}{8}$ tsp. ground black pepper

2 TB. reduced-fat ricotta cheese

1. Over medium-high heat, bring $\frac{1}{4}$ cup water and onion to a boil in a small nonstick skillet. Cover and cook until the onion is slightly softened. Uncover and continue cooking until the water has evaporated.

2. Drizzle in oil and stir until the pan is coated. Cook, stirring regularly, until onion starts to brown.

3. Pour in egg substitute and reduce to low-medium heat, stirring regularly until the egg starts to set. Continue cooking, lifting the edges so the uncooked egg will flow underneath, until nearly done.

4. Reduce heat, and then sprinkle herbs, salt, and pepper over top, then spoon on ricotta.

5. Cover and cook until the egg is done and cheese is hot.

Greek Chicken Salad

Feta cheese livens up this protein-packed salad with a deep, rich flavor.

Yield:	Prep time:	Cook time:	Serving size:
2 servings	10 minutes	N/A	3 cups

Each serving has:
350 calories
20 g fat
10 g carbohydrates
30 g protein

2 TB. extra-virgin olive oil

1 TB. fresh dill

$\frac{1}{3}$ cup red wine vinegar

$\frac{1}{4}$ tsp. salt

$\frac{1}{4}$ tsp. freshly ground black pepper

1 tsp. garlic powder

12 oz. cooked chicken breast, chopped

6 cups romaine lettuce

2 tomatoes, chopped

1 cucumber, peeled and chopped

$\frac{1}{2}$ cup red onion, chopped

$\frac{1}{2}$ cup black olives, sliced

$\frac{1}{2}$ cup feta cheese, crumbled

1. Combine oil, dill, vinegar, salt, pepper, and garlic powder in large bowl. Add chicken, lettuce, tomatoes, cucumber, onion, olives, and feta. Toss before serving in 3-cup portions.

Sweet Grilled Chicken

Satisfy your protein needs and your sweet tooth with this grilled chicken recipe.

Yield:	Prep time:	Cook time:	Serving size:
4 servings	1 hour	20 minutes	1 chicken breast

Each serving has:
150 calories
4 g fat
2 g carbohydrates
30 g protein

$\frac{1}{2}$ tsp. salt	2 tsp. dry mustard
$\frac{1}{4}$ tsp. freshly ground black pepper	2 tsp. light brown sugar
1 tsp. onion powder	4 (6-oz.) boneless, skinless chicken breasts

1. Combine salt, pepper, onion powder, dry mustard, and brown sugar in bowl.

2. Coat chicken with rub and let sit in refrigerator for 1 hour before grilling.

3. Grill chicken on medium-high, turning once.

Lemon Shrimp & Garlic Vegetables

Lemon and garlic take away any fishy bitterness and spice up this vitamin and mineral packed meal.

Yield:	Prep time:	Cook time:	Serving size:
4 servings	30 minutes	10-12 minutes	$\frac{1}{4}$ preparation

Each serving has:
250 calories
6 g fat
15 g carbohydrates
25 g protein

2 tsp. plus 2 tsp. extra-virgin olive oil

2 large red bell peppers, diced

2 lbs. asparagus, trimmed and cut into 1-inch lengths

2 tsp. freshly grated lemon zest

$\frac{1}{4}$ tsp. plus $\frac{1}{4}$ tsp. salt

5 cloves garlic, minced

1 lb. raw shrimp, peeled

1 cup reduced-sodium chicken broth

1 tsp. cornstarch

2 TB. lemon juice

2 TB. chopped fresh parsley

1. Heat 2 teaspoons oil in nonstick skillet over medium heat and add peppers, asparagus, zest, and $\frac{1}{4}$ teaspoon salt, stirring occasionally until vegetables are just softened. Transfer to bowl and cover to keep warm.

2. Add remaining oil and garlic to pan and cook for 30 seconds before adding shrimp. Cook for 1 minute.

3. Combine broth and cornstarch in small bowl, whisk until smooth, and add to pan with remaining salt. Cook, stirring occasionally, until sauce thickens and shrimp are pink. Remove shrimp from heat and stir in lemon juice and parsley.

4. Serve shrimp and sauce over the vegetables and divide evenly between four plates.

Thai Beef Salad

Thanks to the lime and mint, this beef salad offers rich, unique flavor with every bite.

Yield:	Prep time:	Cook time:	Serving size:
4 servings	12 hours	20 minutes	4 oz.

Each serving has:
250 calories
15 g fat
5 g carbohydrates
25 g protein

1 lb. sirloin steak, trimmed of visible fat

1 TB. reduced-sodium soy sauce

½ tsp. freshly ground black pepper

2 scallions, cut into 1-inch pieces

Zest of 1 lime

3 TB. lime juice

½ tsp. sugar

¼ tsp. crushed red pepper

1½ TB. fish sauce

4 cups frisée or curly endive, torn

2 cups red leaf lettuce, torn

2 TB. chopped fresh mint

2 TB. untoasted sesame oil or canola oil

1. Rub steak with soy sauce and black pepper and place on baking sheet. Broil, turning once, until cooked to desired level of doneness. Let sit five minutes, then slice.

2. Mix scallions, lime zest and juice, sugar, crushed red pepper, and fish sauce in dish and place sliced steak in marinade. Coat completely, then cover and refrigerate overnight.

3. Place frisée, mint, and lettuce in salad bowl before serving. Add steak and marinade, drizzle with oil, toss, and serve in 2-cup portions.

Soy-Broiled Salmon

Honey and vinegar combine to sweeten this salmon dish.

Yield:	Prep time:	Cook time:	Serving size:
4 servings	25 minutes	10-12 minutes	4 oz. salmon

Each serving has:
240 calories
15 g fat
5 g carbohydrates
20 g protein

2 TB. soy sauce	1 tsp. minced fresh ginger
1 TB. rice vinegar	1 lb. salmon fillet, skinned, divided
1 TB. honey	into four pieces
1 scallion, minced	1 tsp. sesame seeds, toasted

1. Combine soy sauce, vinegar, honey, scallion, and ginger in bowl and mix well.

2. In a sealable plastic bag, combine salmon with 3 tablespoons of sauce and marinate for 20 minutes in the refrigerator.

3. Preheat broiler and line baking pan with foil coated with cooking spray. Move salmon to pan, skin-side down, and broil 6 inches away from heat source until cooked.

4. Drizzle salmon with remaining sauce and top with sesame seeds.

Grilled Pork Tenderloin

Grilling with sugar and cayenne gives you a spicy, sweet flavor that helps the tenderloin practically melt in your mouth.

Yield:	Prep time:	Cook time:	Serving size:
Varies	1-3 hours	8-12 minutes	4 oz. pork

Each serving has:
130 calories
5 g fat
0 g carbohydrates
20 g protein

$\frac{1}{4}$ cup soy sauce

2 TB. sugar

1 garlic clove, minced

1 cayenne chile pepper, seeded and minced

1 TB. fresh ginger, finely grated

1 TB. toasted sesame oil

1$\frac{1}{2}$ lb. pork tenderloin, trimmed, cut into 1-inch-thick medallions

1. Combine soy sauce and sugar in bowl until sugar dissolves. Add garlic, chile, ginger, and oil and mix.

2. Place pork in sealable plastic bag and add marinade, rotating bag to coat medallions. Refrigerate for 1 to 3 hours, turning once.

3. Over medium heat, grill medallions until cooked through.

Zesty Tuna Steak

Ginger and honey give this tuna a zing that starts with spice and finishes smooth.

Yield:	Prep time:	Cook time:	Serving size:
4 servings	3 hours	4-6 minutes	1 steak

Each serving has:
260 calories
10 g fat
2 g carbohydrates
40 g protein

½ cup soy sauce	2 garlic cloves, minced
¼ cup freshly squeezed orange juice	1 tsp. cornstarch
¼ cup honey	2 TB. sesame oil
1 tsp. fresh ginger, crushed	4 (6-oz.) tuna steaks

1. Combine soy sauce, orange juice, sesame oil, honey, ginger, garlic, and cornstarch in sealable plastic bag and add tuna steaks. Marinate for 3 hours in refrigerator.

2. Grill over medium-high heat until outside is browned.

Vegan Tempeh Burgers

No-meat protein can be plenty flavorful, and this pineapple-infused tempeh dish proves it with a subtle sweetness.

Yield:	Prep time:	Cook time:	Serving size:
4 patties	35 minutes	5-8 minutes	1 patty

Each serving has:
250 calories
11 g fat
15 g carbohydrates
25 g protein

1 lb. tempeh	2 TB. white wine
$\frac{1}{4}$ cup soy sauce	2 cloves garlic, minced
$\frac{1}{4}$ cup pineapple juice	1 TB. ginger, grated
$\frac{1}{2}$ tsp. white pepper	Pinch of red pepper flakes, or to taste

1. Cut tempeh into four even patties.

2. Mix soy sauce, pineapple juice, white pepper, white wine, garlic, ginger, and red pepper flakes together in a large bowl to form a marinade and place patties in mix. Ensure marinade fully coats each patty by turning. Let sit 30 minutes.

3. Grill on medium-high heat, turning halfway through cooking.

Index

A

Ab Lean, 56
abdominal muscle training, 93-95
  Abs and Obliques workout (9), 160
  Arms, Abs, Lower Back/Hips workout (20), 170
  Arms and Abdominals workout (3), 158
  Ball Crunches, 96
  Core workout (22), 172
  Core workout (30), 181
  Core workout (34), 185
  Couch Lifts, 100
  Couch Rolls, 101
  Elevated Side Planks, 106
  Flat Planks, 103
  Hanging Knee Bends, 102
  Hanging Leg Raises, 102
  Knee Bends, 99
  Leg Lifts, 98
  Legs and Abs workout (17), 167
  Medicine Ball Sit-Ups, 108
  Medicine Ball Turns, 109
  Medicine Chin Sit-Ups, 109
  myths, 94-95
  Plank Lifts, 104
  Push-Up Walk-Outs, 107
  Rotating Crunches, 97
  Rotating Planks, 107
  Scissor Kicks, 99
  Shoulders, Abs and Obliques workout (13), 163
  Side Planks, 105
  Single-Knee Bends, 100
  Standard Crunches, 96
  Tall Planks, 103
  V-Ups, 101
  Vertical Crunches, 98
  Walking Planks, 106
Abs and Obliques workout (9), 160
allicin, 22
Alternating Leg Raise Push-Ups, 76
antioxidants, 21-22
Arm Lifts, 110
arms
  Arms, Abs, Lower Back/Hips workout (20), 170
  Arms and Abdominals workout (3), 158
  Arms and Back workout (12), 162
  Arms and Back workout (24), 174
  Arms workout (27), 178
  Cable Curls, 70
  Cable Hammer Curls, 70
  Chest and Arms workout (31), 182

Chest and Arms workout (35), 186

Medicine Ball Arm Curls, 73

Medicine Ball Triceps Extensions, 73

Overhead Extensions, 72

Shoulders and Arms workout (16), 166

Triceps Cable Extensions, 71

Triceps Dips, 71

Triceps Push-Ups, 72

Arms, Abs, Lower Back/Hips workout (20), 170

Arms and Abdominals workout (3), 158

Arms and Back workout (12), 162

Arms and Back workout (24), 174

Arms workout (27), 178

artificial sweeteners, 26

B

back

Arms, Abs, Lower Back/Hips workout (20), 170

Arms and Back workout (12), 162

Arms and Back workout (24), 174

Back and Obliques workout (18), 168

Back workout (5), 158

Cable Column Rows, 90

Exercise Ball Back Squeeze, 86

Lower Back Stretch, 59

Lying Arm Raises (Front), 88

Lying Arm Raises (Side), 88

Medicine Ball Rows, 89

One-Hand Table Pull, 87

Shoulders and Back workout (8), 159

Shoulders and Back workout (29), 180

Shoulders and Back workout (33), 184

Table Pull, 87

Back and Obliques workout (18), 168

Back workout (5), 158

bacteria, healthy, 22

Ball Crunches, 96

Beginning Chest workout (2), 157

Beginning Legs workout (1), 157

beverages, 21-28

bicep muscles

Biceps Stretch, 51

Cable Curls, 70

Cable Hammer Curls, 70

Medicine Ball Arm Curls, 73

Body Twists, 148

bouncing, stretching, 48

breakfast, 37

Bridges, 113

Butt Kicking, 144

Butterfly Stretch, 58

C

Cable Chest Presses, 79

Cable Column Rows, 90

Cable Curls, 70

Cable Hammer Curls, 70

Cable Oblique Bends, 108

Cable Overhead Presses, 80

Cable Post Flies, 79

caffeine, 21

calf muscles

Calf Raises on a Stair, 135

Chest and Calves workout (15), 165

One-Leg Calf Raises, 136

stretches, 66-67

Calf Raises on a Stair, 135

calories
    fat loss, 29
    food labels, 24
    muscle gain, 30
    needs, 29
capsaicin, 22
carbohydrates, 18-19
    food labels, 25
cardiovascular exercise, 139-142
    avoiding boredom, 141-142
    benefits, 139-140
    Body Twists, 148
    Butt Kicking, 144
    circuits, 187-190
    Crossovers, 146
    Dual Squats, 146
    High Knees, 144
    Hop Jumps, 152
    Jumping Jacks, 148
    Knee Jumps, 151
    Long Leaps, 147
    Medicine Ball Overhead Throws, 150
    Medicine Ball Rear Throws, 151
    Medicine Ball Sprints, 150
    Mountain Climbers, 149
    Push-Up U-Jump, 149
    Side Steps, 147
    Ski Jumps, 145
    Star Jumps, 143
    Star Picker, 143
    steady-state, 142
    target heart rate, 141
    Toe Kicks, 145
    versus weight training, 8
casein protein, 198
Celiac disease, 28
Chair Squats, 126

chest, 74
    Alternating Leg Raise Push-Ups, 76
    Beginning Chest workout (2), 157
    Cable Chest Presses, 79
    Cable Post Flies, 79
    Chest and Arms workout (31), 182
    Chest and Arms workout (35), 186
    Chest and Calves workout (15), 165
    Chest and Shoulders workout (10), 160
    Chest and Shoulders workout (19), 169
    Chest and Shoulders workout (23), 173
    Chest and Triceps workout (7), 159
    Chest workout (26), 177
    Decline Push-Ups, 75
    Dip Push-Ups, 77
    Exercise Ball Push-Ups, 76
    Incline Push-Ups, 75
    One-Hand Medicine Ball Push-Ups, 78
    Plyometric Push-Ups, 77
    Two-Hand Medicine Ball Push-Ups, 78
Chest and Arms workout (31), 182
Chest and Arms workout (35), 186
Chest and Calves workout (15), 165
Chest and Shoulders workout (10), 160
Chest and Shoulders workout (19), 169
Chest and Shoulders workout (23), 173
Chest and Triceps workout (7), 159
Chest Stretch on Wall, 50

Chest Stretch on Wall 2, 51
Chest workout (26), 177
chewing gum, 33
cholesterol, food labels, 25
chondroitin, 196
circuits (cardio), 187-190
Close-Knee Squats, 122
coenzyme Q-10, 197
coffee, 21-22
concentrates, protein, 198
core training, 93-95
   Abs and Obliques workout (9), 160
   Arm Lifts, 110
   Arms, Abs, Lower Back/Hips
     workout (20), 170
   Arms and Abdominals workout
     (3), 158
   Back and Obliques workout (18),
     168
   Ball Crunches, 96
   Bridges, 113
   Cable Oblique Bends, 108
   Core workout (22), 172
   Core workout (30), 181
   Core workout (34), 185
   Couch Lifts, 100
   Couch Rolls, 101
   Elevated Side Planks, 106
   Flat Planks, 103
   Hanging Knee Bends, 102
   Hanging Leg Raises, 102
   Hip Draws, 115
   Hip Turns, 116
   Hip Twists, 114
   Knee Bends, 99
   Leg Lifts, 98, 111
   Leg Presses, 112
   Leg Sways, 112
   Legs and Abs workout (17), 167

Medicine Ball Sit-Ups, 108
Medicine Ball Turns, 109
Medicine Chin Sit-Ups, 109
   myths, 94-95
   Plank Lifts, 104
   Push-Up Walk-Outs, 107
   Rotating Crunches, 97
   Rotating Planks, 107
   Scissor Kicks, 99
   Shoulders, Abs and Obliques
     workout (13), 163
   Side Leg Lifts, 115
   Side Planks, 105
   Single-Knee Bends, 100
   Standard Crunches, 96
   Tall Planks, 103
   V-Ups, 101
   Vertical Crunches, 98
   Walking Planks, 106
core stretches, 56
   Ab Lean, 56
   Butterfly Stretch, 58
   Groin Stretch, 60
   Hip Flexor Stretch, 57
   Hip Rotations, 57
   Hip Stretch, 60
   Inner Thigh Stretch, 59
   Lower Back Stretch, 59
   Seated Hip Stretch, 61
   Twisting Hip Stretch, 58
Core workout (22), 172
Core workout (30), 181
Core workout (34), 185
Couch Lifts, 100
Couch Rolls, 101
creatine, 197
Cross Body Stretch, 52
Cross-Leg Hamstring, 65
Crossovers, 146

crunches
  Ball, 96
  Rotating, 97
  Standard, 96
  Vertical, 98
curls
  Cable Curls, 70
  Cable Hammer Curls, 70
  Exercise Hamstring Curls, 133
  Medicine Ball Arm Curls, 73

D

Decline Push-Ups, 75
dehydration, 20, 33
Diamond Push-Ups, 84
diet, 3, 20
  caloric needs, 29
  calories, 29-30
  coffee, 21-22
  costs, 33-36
  energy-boosting foods, 22
  food cravings, 31-33
  food labels, 24-28
  foods to avoid, 28-29
  frozen vegetables, 23
  health-boosting foods, 22
  immunity-boosting foods, 22
  joint relief foods, 22
  junk food, 11
  meal times, 37-38
  metabolism-boosting foods, 22
  negative-calories foods, 23
  nutrition, 15-20
  personal food logs, 38-45
  protein shake, 197-199
  shopping lists, 34-36
  snacking, 30-31
  sports drinks, 23-24
  supplements, 194-197

tea, 20
  versus lifestyle, 15-17
Dip Push-Ups, 77
drop sets, 176
Dual Squats, 146
dynamic stretching, 48

E

Elevated Bridges, 131
Elevated Hamstring Stretch, 65
Elevated Side Planks, 106
energy-boosting foods, 22
Exercise Ball Back Squeeze, 86
Exercise Ball Hamstring Curls, 133
Exercise Ball Push-Ups, 76
Exercise Ball Wall Squats, 121

F

Facedown Quadriceps Stretch, 63
failure, workouts, 176
fat burners, 196
fat-loss calories, 29
fats, 18-19
  food labels, 24
  trans, 25
fibers, 19-20
Flat Planks, 103
food logs, 38-45
foods
  energy-boosting, 22
  frozen vegetables, 23
  health-boosting, 22
  immunity-boosting, 22
  joint relief, 22
  metabolism-boosting, 22
  negative-calorie, 23
  reading labels, 24-28

footwear, 9-10
Forearm Stretch, 54
Forearm Stretch 2, 55
fresh vegetables, versus frozen, 23
Front Laterals, 82
front-label claims, food labels, 26-28
fruits, 19-20

G

garlic, 22
genetic predispositions, 10-12
glucosamine, 196
gluten-free foods, 28
grains, 26
green tea, 20-21
Groin Stretch, 60
gym-free training, 7

H

Half Bridges, 129
Hamstring Leans, 63, 133
Hamstring Lifts, 132
hamstring muscles
    Elevated Bridges, 131
    Exercise Ball Hamstring Curls,
        133
    Half Bridges, 129
    Hamstring Leans, 63, 133
    Hamstring Lifts, 132
    Medicine Ball Lifts, 134
    One-Leg Chair Dips, 129
    One-Leg Elevated Bridges, 130
    One-Leg Half Bridges, 130
    stretches, 63-65
Hand Walks, 83

Hanging Knee Bends, 102
Hanging Leg Raises, 102
health-boosting foods, 22
healthy bacteria, 22
heart rate, cardiovascular exercise,
    141
heel cushions, shoes, 9-10
High Knees, 144
high-fructose corn syrup, 28
Hip Draws, 115
Hip Flexor Stretch, 57
Hip Rotations, 57
Hip Stretch, 60
hip stretches
    Butterfly Stretch, 58
    Groin Stretch, 60
    Hip Flexor Stretch, 57
    Hip Rotations, 57
    Hip Stretch, 60
    Inner Thigh Stretch, 59
    Serated Hip Stretch, 61
    Twisting Hip Stretch, 58
Hip Turns, 116
Hip Twists, 114
Hop Jumps, 152
hot peppers, 22
hydration, 33
hydrogenated oil, 28

I

immunity-boosting foods, 22, 27
Incline Push-Ups, 75
ingredients, food labels, 26
Inner Thigh Stretch, 59
insoluble fiber, 20
isolates, protein, 198

J

joint relief, foods, 22
Journal of Biological Chemistry, 22
journals, food, 38-45
Jumping Jacks, 148
junk food, avoiding, 11

K

kitchens, readying, 5
Knee Bends, 99
Knee Drops, 123
Knee Jumps, 151
Knee Pull, 64

L

labels, food, reading, 24-28
Lean Stretch, 53
Leaning Neck Stretch, 50
Leaning Squats, 127
Leg Lifts, 98, 111
Leg Presses, 112
legs
    Beginning Legs workout (1), 157
    Calf Raises on a Stair, 135
    Chair Squats, 126
    Chest and Calves workout (15),
      165
    Close-Knee Squats, 122
    Elevated Bridges, 131
    Exercise Ball Hamstring Curls,
      133
    Exercise Ball Wall Squats, 121
    Half Bridges, 129
    Hamstring Leans, 133
    Hamstring Lifts, 132
    Knee Drops, 123

Leaning Squats, 127
Legs and Abs workout (17), 167
Legs workout (11), 161
Legs workout (21), 171
Legs workout (32), 183
Lower Body workout (6), 159
Lower Body workout (14), 164
Lower Body workout (25), 175-176
Lower Body workout (28), 179
Lunges, 124
Medicine Ball Lifts, 134
Medicine Ball Squat-Presses, 128
One-Leg Calf Raises, 136
One-Leg Chair Dips, 129
One-Leg Chair Squats, 124, 126
One-Leg Elevated Bridges, 130
One-Leg Half Bridges, 130
Rotating Lunges, 127
Squat Holds, 121
Squat Jumps, 125
Squats, 120
Step-Ups, 125
Leg Sways, 112
Legs and Abs workout (17), 167
Legs workout (11), 161
Legs workout (21), 171
Legs workout (32), 183
Lifted Hamstring Stretch, 66
live active cultures, yogurt, 22
logs, food, 38-45
Long Leaps, 147
Lower Back Stretch, 59
lower body stretches, 61-67
lower body training, 119
    Calf Raises on a Stair, 135
    Chair Squats, 126
    Close-Knee Squats, 122
    Elevated Bridges, 131
    Exercise Ball Hamstring Curls,
      133

Exercise Ball Wall Squats, 121
Half Bridges, 129
Hamstring Leans, 133
Hamstring Lifts, 132
Knee Drops, 123
Leaning Squats, 127
Lunges, 124
Medicine Ball Lifts, 134
Medicine Ball Squat-Presses, 128
One-Leg Calf Raises, 136
One-Leg Chair Dips, 129
One-Leg Chair Squats, 124-126
One-Leg Elevated Bridges, 130
One-Leg Half Bridges, 130
Rotating Lunges, 127
Squat Holds, 121
Squat Jumps, 125
Squats, 120
Step-Ups, 125
Lower Body workout (6), 159
Lower Body workout (14), 164
Lower Body workout (25), 175-176
Lower Body workout (28), 179
Lunges, 124
Lying Arm Raises (Front), 88
Lying Arm Raises (Side), 88

M

mass, muscle training, 8
maximum heart rate (MHR), 141
meal times, 37-38
Medicine Ball Arm Curls, 73
Medicine Ball Circles, 85
Medicine Ball Lifts, 134
Medicine Ball Overhead Throws, 150
Medicine Ball Rear Throws, 151
Medicine Ball Rows, 89
Medicine Ball Sit-Ups, 108
Medicine Ball Sprints, 150

Medicine Ball Squat-Presses, 128
Medicine Ball Triceps Extensions, 73
Medicine Ball Turns, 109
Medicine Chin Sit-Ups, 109
mental health, improving, 140
metabolism-boosting foods, 22
Metamucil, 19
methylsulfonylmethane (MSM), 197
MHR (maximum heart rate), 141
modified food starch, 28
Mom's Monthly, 195
Mountain Climbers, 149
MSM (methylsulfonylmethane), 197
multigrain foods, 26
multivitamins, 196
muscle-gain calories, 30
Muscular Development, 195
myths, core training, 94-95

N

natural claims, food labels, 26
negative-calorie foods, 23
nutrition, 15-20
    caloric needs, 29
    calories, 29-30
    carbohydrates, 18-19
    coffee, 21-22
    energy-boosting foods, 22
    fats, 18-19
    fibers, 19-20
    food labels, 24-28
    foods to avoid, 28-29
    frozen vegetables, 23
    fruits, 19-20
    health-boosting foods, 22
    immunity-boosting foods, 22
    joint relief foods, 22
    metabolism-boosting foods, 22
    negative-calorie foods, 23

protein, 18-19
snacking, 30-31
sports drinks, 23-24
supplements, 195-199
tea, 20
vegetables, 19-20
nutrition panel, food labels, 24

O

oblique muscle training, 93-95
  Abs and Obliques workout (9), 160
  Back and Obliques workout (18),
    168
  Ball Crunches, 96
  Cable Oblique Bends, 108
  Core workout (22), 172
  Couch Lifts, 100
  Couch Rolls, 101
  Elevated Side Planks, 106
  Flat Planks, 103
  Hanging Knee Bends, 102
  Hanging Leg Raises, 102
  Knee Bends, 99
  Leg Lifts, 98
  Medicine Ball Sit-Ups, 108
  Medicine Ball Turns, 109
  Medicine Chin Sit-Ups, 109
  myths, 94-95
  Plank Lifts, 104
  Push-Up Walk-Outs, 107
  Rotating Crunches, 97
  Rotating Planks, 107
  Scissor Kicks, 99
  Shoulders, Abs and Obliques
    workout (13), 163
  Side Planks, 105
  Single-Knee Bends, 100
  Standard Crunches, 96
  stretches, 56
  Tall Planks, 103
  Vertical Crunches, 98
  V-Ups, 101
  Walking Planks, 106
One-Hand Medicine Ball Push-Ups,
  78
One-Hand Table Pull, 87
One-Leg Calf Raises, 136
One-Leg Chair Dips, 129
One-Leg Chair Squats, 124-126
One-Leg Elevated Bridges, 130
One-Leg Half Bridges, 130
organic claims, food labels, 27
Overhead Extensions, 72
Overhead Medicine Ball Raises, 85
overtraining risks, 194

P

pain, 9
  stretching, 48
partially hydrogenated oil, 28
partials, 176
pectoral muscles
  Alternating Leg Raise Push-Ups,
    76
  Cable Chest Presses, 79
  Cable Post Flies, 79
  Decline Push-Ups, 75
  Dip Push-Ups, 77
  Exercise Ball Push-Ups, 76
  Incline Push-Ups, 75
  One-Hand Medicine Ball Push-
    Ups, 78
  Plyometric Push-Ups, 77
  Two-Hand Medicine Ball Push-
    Ups, 78
personal food logs, 38-45
Plank Lifts, 104

planks
    Elevated Side Planks, 106
    Flat Planks, 103
    Plank Lifts, 104
    Rotating Planks, 107
    Side Planks, 105
    Tall Planks, 103
    Walking Plank, 84
    Walking Planks, 106
Plyometric Push-Ups, 77
post-workout meals, 38
potassium, food labels, 25
predispositions, genetics, 10-12
pre-workout meals, 38
progress, recording, 7
protein, 18-19
    food labels, 25
    shakes, 197-199
push-ups
    Alternating Leg Raise Push-Ups,
        76
    Decline Push-Ups, 75
    Dip Push-Ups, 77
    Exercise Ball Push-Ups, 76
    Incline Push-Ups, 75
    One-Hand Medicine Ball Push-
        Ups, 78
    Polymetric Push-Ups, 77
    Push-Up U-Jump, 149
    Push-Up Walk-Outs, 107
    Shoulder Push-Ups, 80
    Triceps Push-Ups, 72
    Two-Hand Medicine Ball Push-
        Ups, 78
Push-Up U-Jump, 149
Push-Up Walk-Outs, 107

Q

quadricep muscles
    Chair Squats, 126
    Close-Knee Squats, 122
    Exercise Ball Wall Squats, 121
    Facedown Quadriceps Stretch, 63
    Knee Drops, 123
    Leaning Squats, 127
    Lunges, 124
    Medicine Ball Squat-Presses, 128
    One-Leg Chair Squats, 124-126
    Rotating Lunges, 127
    Seated Quadriceps Stretch, 62
    Squat Holds, 121
    Squat Jumps, 125
    Squats, 120
    Standing Quadriceps Stretch, 62
    Step-Ups, 125

R

Raised Triceps Stretch, 52
raises
    Hanging Leg Raises, 102
    Lying Arm Raises (Front), 88
    Lying Arm Raises (Side), 88
    Overhead Medicine Ball Raises, 85
reading
    food labels, 24-28
reality television shows, 4-5
Rear Laterals, 83
recovery, 193-194
refined grains, 26
rest and recovery, 193-194
restaurants
    menu choices, 6
Rotating Crunches, 97
Rotating Lunges, 127

Rotating Planks, 107
routines (cardio), 187-190

S

safety, stretching, 49
Scissor Kicks, 99
sea salt, 27
Seated Forearm Stretch, 55
Seated Hamstring Stretch, 64
Seated Hip Stretch, 61
Seated Quadriceps Stretch, 62
serving sizes, food labels, 24
shoes, 9-10
shopping list, 34-36
Shoulder Push-Ups, 80
shoulders
    Back workout (5), 158
    Cable Overhead Presses, 80
    Chest and Shoulders (10), 160
    Chest and Shoulders workout (19),
      169
    Chest and Shoulders workout (23),
      173
    Diamond Push-Ups, 84
    Front Laterals, 82
    Hand Walks, 83
    Medicine Ball Circles, 85
    Overhead Medicine Ball Raises, 85
    Rear Laterals, 83
    Shoulder Push-Ups, 80
    Shoulders, Abs and Obliques
      workout (13), 163
    Shoulders and Arms workout (16),
      166
    Shoulders and Back workout (8),
      159
    Shoulders and Back workout (29),
      180

    Shoulders and Back workout (33),
      184
    Shoulders workout (4), 158
    Side Laterals, 81
    Walking Plank, 84
Shoulders, Abs and Obliques workout
  (13), 163
Shoulders and Arms workout (16),
  166
Shoulders and Back workout (8), 159
Shoulders and Back workout (29), 180
Shoulders and Back workout (33), 184
Shoulders workout (4), 158
Side Laterals, 81
Side Leg Lifts, 115
Side Planks, 105
Side Steps, 147
Single-Knee Bends, 100
Ski Jumps, 145
sleep hygiene, importance, 193-194
snacking, 30-31
sodium, 25-27
soluble fiber, 19
soy protein, 198
sports drinks versus water, 23-24
spot toning, 8
Squat Holds, 121
Squat Jumps, 125
squats
    Chair Squats, 126
    Close Knee Squats, 122
    Dual Squats, 146
    Exercise Ball Wall Squats, 121
    Leaning Squats, 127
    One-Leg Chair Squats, 124-126
    Squat Holds, 121
    Squat Jumps, 125
    Squats, 120
Squats, 120

Standard Crunches, 96
Standing Quadriceps Stretch, 62
Star Jumps, 143
Star Picker, 143
static stretching, 48
steady-state cardiovascular exercise, 142
Step-Ups, 125
Streamline Stretch, 54
stretching, 47
   attire, 48
   benefits, 48
   bouncing, 48
   core, 56-61
   duration, 49
   dynamic, 48
   frequency, 49
   importance, 47-48
   lower body, 61-67
   pain, 48
   safety, 49
   static, 48
   upper body, 49-55
   warm-Up, 48
sucralose, 26
supersets, 176
supplements, 194
   advertisements, 195
   effective, 196-197
   facts, 195-196
   protein shakes, 197-199
sweeteners, artificial, 26

T

Table Pull, 87
table salt, 27
Tall Planks, 103
target heart rate, cardiovascular exercise, 141

tea, 20
testosterone, 8
thermogenics, 196
Toe Kicks, 145
toning, 8
toning shoes, 9
Towel Stretch, 53
trans fats, 25, 28
tricep muscles
   Chest and Triceps workout (7), 159
   Medicine Ball Triceps Extensions, 73
   Overhead Extensions, 72
   Triceps Cable Extensions, 71
   Triceps Dips, 71
   Triceps Push-Ups, 72
Triceps Cable Extensions, 71
Triceps Dips, 71
Triceps Push-Ups, 72
turmeric, 22
Twisting Hip Stretch, 58
Two-Hand Medicine Ball Push-Ups, 78

U–V

upper body stretches, 49
   Biceps Stretch, 51
   Chest Stretch on Wall, 50
   Chest Stretch on Wall 2, 51
   Cross Body Stretch, 52
   Forearm Stretch, 54
   Forearm Stretch 2, 55
   Lean Stretch, 53
   Leaning Neck Stretch, 50
   Raised Triceps Stretch, 52
   Seated Forearm Stretch, 55
   Streamline Stretch, 54
   Towel Stretch, 53

upper body training, 69
  arms, 69
    Cable Curls, 70
    Cable Hammer Curls, 70
    Medicine Ball Arm Curls, 73
    Medicine Ball Triceps
      Extensions, 73
    Overhead Extensions, 72
    Triceps Cable Extensions, 71
    Triceps Dips, 71
    Triceps Push-Ups, 72
  back, 86
    Cable Column Rows, 90
    Exercise Ball Back Squeeze, 86
    Lying Arm Raises (Front), 88
    Lying Arm Raises (Side), 88
    Medicine Ball Rows, 89
    One-Hand Table Pull, 87
    Table Pull, 87
  chest, 74
    Alternating Leg Raise Push-
      Ups, 76
    Cable Chest Presses, 79
    Cable Post Flies, 79
    Decline Push-Ups, 75
    Dip Push-Ups, 77
    Exercise Ball Push-Ups, 76
    Incline Push-Ups, 75
    One-Hand Medicine Ball Push-
      Ups, 78
    Plyometric Push-Ups, 77
    Two-Hand Medicine Ball
      Push-Ups, 78
  shoulders, 80-85

V-Ups, 101
vegetables, 19-20
Vertical Crunches, 98
vitamin D, 197

W–X–Y–Z

Walking Plank, 84
Walking Planks, 106
Wall Calf Stretch, 66-67
water versus sports drinks, 23-24
whey protein, 198
whole grains, 26
workouts, 155-157
  See also specific workouts
  cardio circuits, 187-190
  drop sets, 176
  duration, 155-156
  failure, 176
  frequency, 155-156
  supersets, 176

yogurt, 22

Also by Nathan Jendrick

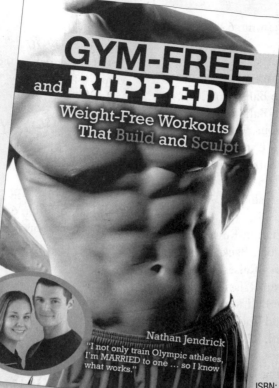

ISBN: 978-1-61564-099-7
$16.95 US/ $19.50 CAN

No gym?
No problem!

Gym-Free and Ripped shows you how to trim and sculpt your body without stepping foot in a gym or blowing your budget on bulky and expensive home machines.

The book includes dozens of exercises, eight weekly workouts, nutrition information, and sample recipes.

ALPHA